Low-Stress Fitness

An Easy-Does-It Exercise Plan For Any Age
Stretching, Walking, Bicycling & Swimming

Millie Brown
Foreword by Bill Rodgers

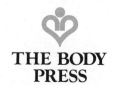

**THE BODY
PRESS**

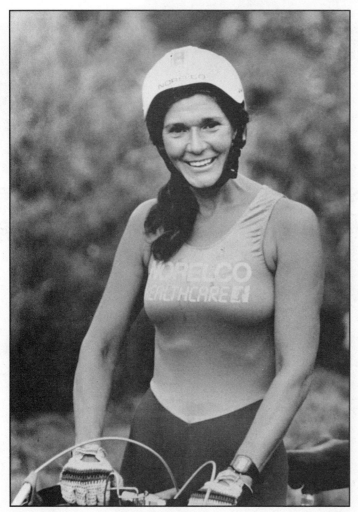

Photo: Bill Travis

Dedication
This book is dedicated to my daughter Chris, my best friend and secretary. Also to my sons Larry and Mark, my father Irv Oeth, my family, friends and the memory of my mother and Aunts Vera and Mildred.

Acknowledgments
The following people have offered encouragement, support and advice: Linda, John and Fred Sammis; Susan Cass; Richard Q. Kress and the Norelco Consumer Products Division; Bob Grant; and the Lancelot in my life.

Published by The Body Press, a division of HPBooks, Inc.
P.O. Box 5367, Tucson, AZ 85703   602/888-2150
ISBN: 0-89586-355-3
Library of Congress Catalog No. 85-80119
© 1985 HPBooks, Inc.
Printed in U.S.A.

Contents

Publisher
Rick Bailey

Editorial Director
Theodore DiSante

Editor
Virginia Fraps Hodge

Art Director
Don Burton

Book Design
Leslie Sinclair

Typography
Cindy Coatsworth,
Michelle Carter

Book Manufacture
Anthony B. Narducci

B&W Photos
Barbara Nitke, Melchior
DiGiacomo, Ed Stiles

Front Cover Photo
© Gregory Gorfkle, 1985. All
rights reserved.

Illustrations
Allan Mogel

Make-up
Eva Polywka

Model
Madonna Christian

Material prepared by
Rutledge Books, a division of
Sammis Publishing
Corporation, 122 E. 25th St.,
New York, NY 10010

Foreword

It's appropriate for Millie Brown to write a book on this subject rather than the usual doctor, coach or professional athlete. Millie developed her fitness level through experience, at an age later than most people would consider trying.

I greatly admire people like Millie. In fact, my favorite athletes are not the world-class ones, but the folks of "average" ability who realize that their fitness is a gift. And I am not alone: A friend of mine who represented the U.S. Olympic team in 1972 was asked at a training clinic who his favorite athlete was. He answered, "My father." His father had recently quit smoking, began running and even completed a marathon.

No amount of money can make you fit, yet fitness is not hard to come by. Certainly our society would benefit from an overall improvement in the fitness level of our citizens. Programs and books like this one—stressing all-around activity—are needed to reach people who think that fitness is for an elite, athletic group, instead of for everyone.

I'm sure that you will be inspired by Millie's own story and feel encouraged by her easy-does-it fitness program. Walking, swimming and bicycling are safe, easy and fun! I believe that some day we will have a society in which feeling fit and healthy is the norm. This book will play a positive role in making that ideal a reality.

Bill Rodgers
Boston, Massachusetts

CHAPTER ONE

A True Beginning

I was moving rapidly toward a watershed birthday, my 40th, bitter in the knowledge that life had bested me. I was divorced, depressed and totally out of shape physically. Worse, I seemed out of prospects.

That's when I turned myself around. I began with the obvious—my physical shape. When that began to improve through a physical-fitness program, my mental state also started improving. But I did it the hard way. I went all-out to competitive extremes that ultimately swept me past marathons and into triathlons.

But what I *learned* in the process of going from a dyspeptic approaching 40 to a triathlon winner is in this book. I hope to persuade all of you who aren't in good shape—emotionally or physically—that there is a way to become stronger, healthier and happier, but without going to the physical extremes I did.

MY PLAN FOR YOU

You can achieve good health with a *low-stress fitness program* using aerobic principles. This is not a now-and-then program, something you do when the urge strikes, but a carefully constructed program free of the physical risks of many other approaches. My program involves no threat of injury to knees or shins, no strained ligaments, no sore back and no damaged tendons.

This program is enjoyable. You will find it fun and something to look forward to each day. Whether you are swimming, walking or cycling, you won't rate progress on how fast or how far you go. You will measure it by the pleasure you have gaining the fitness you really want.

You can begin the program *at any age* and continue on into your 80s. You can follow it alone or in the company of others. *Anyone* with a free hour can use it to improve himself or herself.

Athletes, regardless of age or ability, constantly work on self-improvement. Training helps them avoid feelings of inadequacy. Sports builds their self-confidence and raises their self-esteem. These benefits of physical well-being and improved mental outlook can be yours, too, when you start my low-stress fitness program.

You can be such an "athlete." And you can do it without pressure and without stress.

HOW I BECAME AN IRONWOMAN

It all began for me when I was 38 years old. My life was filled with insecurities and fears. I constantly felt tired. I lacked enthusiasm. I would wake at 6 a.m. and lie in bed worrying about bills, about my mother who had cancer, about how I would manage to send three kids through college. I anguished over being divorced. And it seemed to me that every day I was becoming more susceptible to illness and further despair.

I can't tell you the exact day it happened, but something changed suddenly. One morning instead of staying in bed I got up, dressed and headed for the beach at a fast pace. (I live in Rowayton, Connecticut, a lovely and sleepy village facing Long Island Sound.) Along the way, I paused to do a few stretching exercises I remembered seeing in a magazine. I knew next to nothing about stretching or aerobic principles. What I was doing was instinctive.

The next morning without questioning myself I got up again and took another walk. By the time I returned to my house I had made a rule: Think only positive thoughts while walking.

The Next Step—This self-imposed "training" continued for a while. It wasn't long before my children noticed my improved disposition at breakfast. On my next birthday they gave me a gift certificate for a pair of running shoes.

At the shoe store, the salesman said, "Why don't you enter the Rowayton running race next Saturday?"

I scoffed. "I've never even run a mile. At my age, run a race? You're out of your mind."

"No I'm not," he insisted. "You walk and jog, don't you? Then you can run. Go ahead. Give it a try."

On my way out of the store, to my surprise, I thought, "Why not?"

My First Race—I walked more than I ran in that first race. It was a three-mile, cross-country event. I got lost once, fell twice and had to make one pit stop in the bushes. The finish line was in the process of being dismantled when I reached it, but I went charging across, my arms in the air, looking and feeling like a winner. I'd finished, hadn't I?

From then on, I was hooked.

But my training to become a runner was anything but scientific. I knew nothing about "target heart rates." If I felt tired or out of breath, I would simply slow down and walk. If I felt pain, I stopped until the pain left.

Every few races, I entered a longer one. It wasn't that I was winning so much as enjoying myself immensely, and I felt a great sense of accomplishment, so I always crossed the finish line smiling.

First Marathon—After one of the longer races a running pal said, "How about if we run together in the New York Marathon?"

Two years earlier, I dreaded each birthday. Now, with my 40th approaching, I was accepting one of the premier running challenges—the New York Marathon, 26.2 miles of urban racing.

Those two previous years of physical activity brought me more than physical fitness. It strengthened my moral fiber. At 38 it didn't occur to me it might be too late to educate my mind as well as discipline my body.

At 40 it dawned on me that I could do just about anything I set my mind to. Certainly if I could run 26.2 miles on the streets of New York, I could find the courage to enroll in college—which is what I did. I mailed in my application for the marathon and signed up for classes at Norwalk Community College. Trembling, I went home and toasted myself with a glass of wine.

I suppose you want to know how I did in the marathon? I did OK, finishing in 4 hours, 50 minutes. The friend who ran with me said, "You act like you're the mayor and all these people came out here to see you." Actually, that *is* how I felt. The part of me that hurt the most after the race was my face—from smiling.

Toward the Triathlon—In my late 20s I had learned to ice skate and worked as an instructor at a skating rink. When I began training for marathon running, I spent a lot of time ice skating at the rink near my home. It was while I was skating that I first heard about triathlon competition. I was interested more in the variety of events than in the demands on its competitors.

My main problem with the triathlon was that I had a fear of the water. Why I entered my first local triathlon—a 1-mile swim, 27-mile bike race and 10-mile run—is anybody's guess. Hooked on running? Hooked on seeing how much my body would suffer? Probably both.

What I lacked in training, I made up for in tenacity. I swam the backstroke so I wouldn't have to put my face in the water. Then I discovered that I was swimming against the tide. Though I swam my best, I couldn't cross the finish

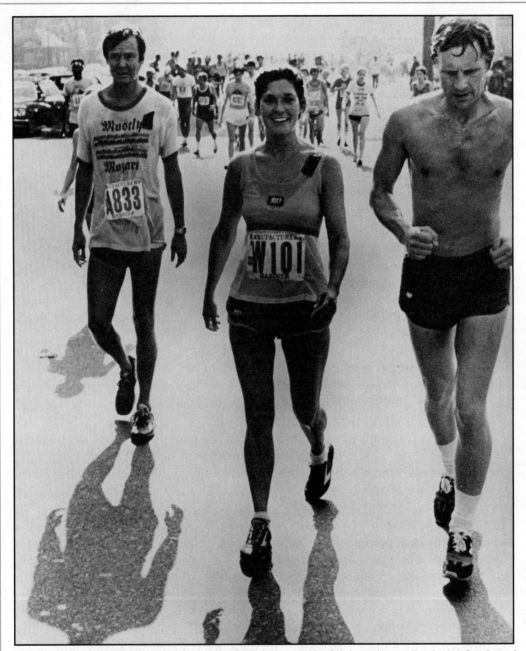

My first New York City Marathon was in 1979. I ran much of it, but also walked a lot. I enjoyed myself for the whole 4 hours and 50 minutes, as you can tell by the smile on my face.

line. Finally, the race officials hauled me out of the water. I pleaded with them to let me go on, but they told me, "We're not losing anyone in this race." They did let me continue in the other events.

I sailed through the hilly bike course and the 10-mile foot race. But I was still unhappy about my failure in the water.

"I'm going back into the water," I announced. Under the supervision of a lifeguard, I did enough laps to finish the mile I had started.

It was in that first triathlon I realized how psyched up athletes can become in competition. Carried away by the pressures and challenges, they take chances and disregard danger signs.

Academic Credentials—I decided then that a classroom study of sports and fitness would be helpful if I was going to train and compete athletically. At that time my local community college offered a certification in athletic coaching, so I signed up for it and every other fitness-related course offered.

Going to class, getting decent grades and finishing races with improved standings were great ego builders. I was definitely feeling good about myself. I was relaxed and about ready to admit that there was an element of happiness in my life. No longer was I saying, "I can't." I substituted "I'll try" or "Why not?"

Iron (wo) man—I found myself daring to dream of larger goals—specifically the so-called Ironman Triathlon. Believe me, it has earned its epithet. It consists of a 2.4-mile swim, a 112-mile bicycle race and a 26.2-mile foot race—all one after the other. Even the time needed between races for change of outfit is charged against the athlete.

If I could be accepted for the Ironman I figured I would have traveled the full route—going from an out-of-shape, despairing divorcée to a top athlete competing in the most demanding competition around.

When you put your body on the line for this kind of event, you try to learn all you can about the sport. Could it be enjoyed or simply endured? When I finally finished my first triathlon, I had to admit that 95% was enjoyable. The fact that at my age I not only entered, but finished, made sports headlines. The following year, ABC-TV cameras followed me in the race.

I was thinking, anything's possible! So I ran a 12-hour race, then a 50-mile race. Since, I've entered 25 triathlons, winning or placing in all but 6. And I've remained relatively injury free, though I now believe that was largely by chance.

A WOMAN'S MIND SET

Training and experience are a lot more important than gender in athletic performance. The difference between male and female physical potential for performance is not as great as was originally believed.

Muscle—The quality of muscle—its contractile properties and ability to exert

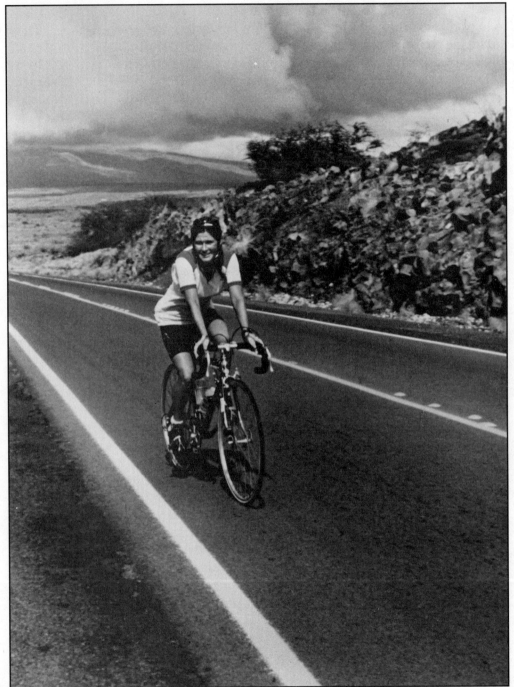

This is from the 112-mile bicycling phase of the first "real" triathlon I entered in 1982. Notice that I'm still smiling!

force—and neuromuscular efficiency are the same in both sexes, according to Dr. Jack Wilmore of the University of Arizona. If a man and a woman are of equal size and have an equal percentage of body fat, they most likely will be equally strong.

With equal opportunity and activity, the gap between physical performances in the sexes could be 10% or less, according to some exercise physiologists. Some researchers believe there is little or no reason to advocate different training programs for men and women.

Injury—Women are no more subject to injury than men. The 10% to 12% more body fat women have provides a built-in protective layer of fat stored between skin and muscle. Body projections are better protected from injury. The extra layer of fat also insulates a woman against cold and makes her more buoyant in water. Women also have advantages over men in ultra-distance and endurance sports because of the extra fat they can burn for energy.

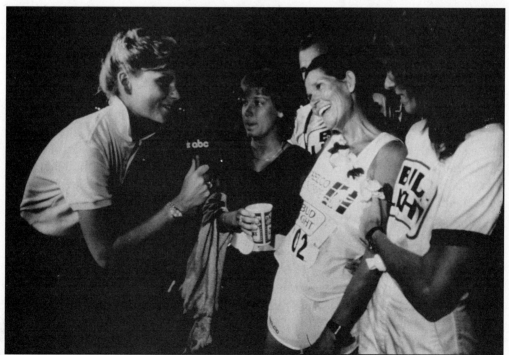

Here, I'm being interviewed by Terri Blair of ABC-TV at the end of the 1983 Ironman in Hawaii. I think I'm telling her about wanting to write a book on low-stress exercise.

More Trends and Stats — Today the number of women beginning to participate in every popular sport far exceeds the number of male newcomers. According to statistics compiled by Sandra Rosenzweig for *Sportsfitness for Women,* "Three out of every five new runners or bicyclists are women, and so are four out of every five baseball and basketball players. Women comprise 49% of all tennis players, 44% of all downhill skiers, 39% of all backpackers, 36% of all squash players, 33% of all high-school athletes, and 30% of all college athletes."

Only in recent years, however, have women trained with the technical guidance, concentration and confidence men have always received. Fortunately, our culture is changing, and the myths concerning woman's frailty are being refuted.

A MAN'S MIND SET

In sports, men have more pressure on them than women do. The cultural attitude is that men need to be tough, strong and fast. Such an attitude makes it much harder for a man to participate in an enjoyable, non-stressful exercise program. The men who choose my low-stress program may have to ignore some of this thinking.

Attitude — I have seen men start a sport but drop out because they felt they were not progressing quickly enough. The time they did spend at it was drudgery because they tried to do too much, too soon.

For example, it requires patience and understanding for a man to enter an aerobic program slowly and easily, rather than to charge into it like a young bull. They should forget the athletic feats of their younger years. Unless you have kept up the sports you did as a young man, you have probably lost conditioning and will risk injury if you do not build up stamina slowly.

I cringe when my high-powered executive friends tell me about company picnics or meetings involving sports events. These intelligent, competitive men, many of whom do not exercise regularly, often challenge their peers to vigorous athletic battles. Bets are placed, adrenalin runs high, prestige and self-esteem are at stake. Unfortunately, competitors flirt with injury.

Women's increased training and acceptance in sports have created difficulties for some men. I have seen men near collapse at the finish line of races muttering, "I wasn't going to let that woman pass me."

Men don't have to be like Tarzan, but they do need to keep fit. Society has placed a different set of expectations on men and women, stereotyping men as competitive and women as passive. But times and cultural attitudes are changing.

Low-Stress Exercise For Men — Swimming, cycling and walking do not require the Herculean body needed for football, the height required for basketball, nor the eye/hand coordination for baseball and racket sports. Many non-athletic boys have become successful athletes at middle age by including aerobics as part of their fitness plans. It's never too late. Age is no deterrent. The abilities and skills can be learned—but it does require patience.

BENEFITS OF REGULAR EXERCISE

You and your health should be the number-one concerns in your life. If they aren't, your life could be shortened considerably. Even modest exercise helps prolong life, according to medical researchers at Harvard and Stanford universities. In a study involving some 17,000 middle-aged and older men, the scientists concluded that Americans should undertake some form of regular exercise, such as brisk walks, to help ward off cardiovascular and pulmonary disease. Dr. Ralph S. Paffenbarger, a visiting professor of epidemiology at Harvard's School of Public Health and a member of Stanford's medical faculty, writes, "This is the first good evidence that people who are active and fit have a longer life span than those who are not."

The report notes that "consistency of habit during nine or more months of the year may be necessary to maintain cardiovascular health." The report appeared in the July 1984 issue of the *Journal of the AMA*.

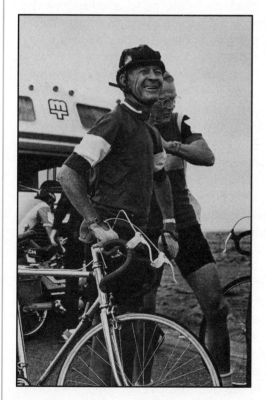

Don't let age be a barrier to fitness. Fred Knoller (the man with the bike) was 89 at the time of this writing and still exercising and competing in bicycle races. You'll learn more about Fred in chapter 7.

Journal editor Dr. Bruce B. Dan comments, "The real discovery of this research is not that people who exercise have strong cardiovascular systems, rather it is that sedentary people have more cardiovascular disease. Sedentary people have shriveled hearts and most of us who do not exercise have atrophied bodies. Since we can now show a direct cause-and-effect relationship between fitness and life span, the message will become much clearer in the minds of most people. We can now prove that large numbers of Americans are dying from sitting on their behinds."

The Role of Blood Pressure—Recent estimates indicate that one in every six adults, or more than 35 million people, have high blood pressure and may be classified as hypertensive. It is one of the most serious and widespread diseases in the United States. People must become more knowledgeable about this "silent killer."

Blood pressure is a measurement of the force exerted by the heart to pump blood through the arteries and the resistance to this flow by blood vessels. The heart contracts and then relaxes, resulting in two levels of blood pressure. The contraction of the heart produces a higher pressure level, termed *systolic*. The relaxation of the heart produces a lower pressure level, termed *diastolic*.

Blood pressure is never constant—it changes according to the needs of the body and may be affected by mental and physical activities. For instance, a higher reading may result from anxiety, physical exertion, smoking, eating or stress.

Also, blood pressure can change day by day or hour by hour, so it is important to monitor and record measurements accurately on a regular basis. It is recommended that blood pressure readings be taken at the same time each day.

High blood pressure has no definitive warning signals or typical symptoms, but regular monitoring can detect high or low blood pressure for early treatment. Because of the normal, daily fluctuations of blood pressure, it is difficult to establish a norm.

While blood pressure varies with mental and physical conditions, it also differs by age, sex, weight and other factors. For adults, systolic pressure readings between 110 and 140 are generally considered normal. Diastolic pressure readings between 70 and 90 are also considered normal.

A home blood-pressure meter should be a part of every home-medicine cabinet. Norelco, for example, has a complete line of blood-pressure meters for home use. Their meters have been extensively tested and have a warranty.

Dr. Erin O'Brien and Professor Kevin O'Malley, authors of *High Blood Pressure,* advocate, "The layman must take some responsibility for prevention and a great deal for management and control of high blood pressure."

Don't check your own blood pressure in lieu of a check-up with a physician. Consider it a supplement. If you are over 30, overweight, have been

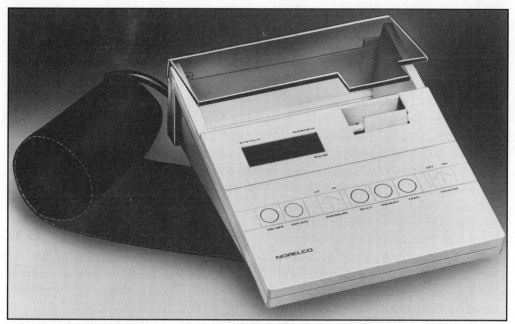

With a Norelco home blood-pressure meter, you can monitor improvements in blood pressure as you become healthier. The illustration below shows different ranges for normal, borderline and hypertense people. Photo and graph courtesy of Norelco Consumer Products Division.

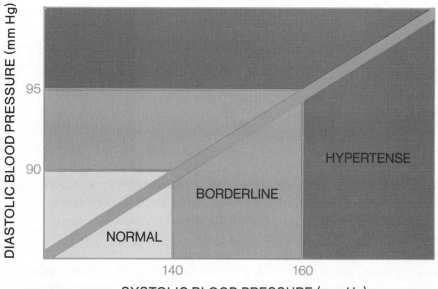

sedentary for several years, are a heavy smoker, use alcohol or drugs, or have any medical problems, you should check with your doctor before embarking on any exercise program—even my low-stress plan. A doctor can tell you if it's necessary to have a physical examination before you start exercising.

Make the Commitment and Reap the Rewards—Dedicate a small part of your day to the pursuit of fitness. Your rewards will be bountiful. You'll feel, look and sleep better. You can improve digestion and your cardiovascular system. You'll have fewer physical complaints, aches and pains, and greater resistance to common illnesses such as colds and the flu.

You will have less anxiety, depression and hypochondria. Your energy will increase and improve along with your self-image and self-confidence. It *is* possible to slow the aging process, lower your pulse rate and lose weight too.

The traditional concept has been that from age 30 on, each year "costs" you a loss of endurance of at least 1%. But typically that level of decline is caused by inactivity. People automatically say, "Oh, you're getting older, so you're losing your endurance." What you are really doing is becoming less active. It has also been observed that athletes who remain active in their later years show less effects of aging.

In 1983 I stopped exercising for two months after some Ironman events. I was burned out, physically and emotionally. I wanted to rest my body completely but found that conditioning was lost very quickly. My period of inactivity caused me to lose much of my strength, power, flexibility, and muscular and cardiovascular endurance. It took months to come back gradually, though emotionally I knew I was still strong and capable. I discovered that the self-confidence and knowledge that I've recently gained from my sports will never leave me.

Dr. Kenneth Cooper says, "Biblically, our bodies are designed to last us 120 years. The reason they don't is not because of a design deficiency, but because of the way we treat our bodies." If you want to live to be 100 or older, you can't just sit around waiting for it to happen!

Psychologists now believe that regular exercise can dramatically slow the progress of many conditions of aging. Age is no impediment to fitness. Older athletes may go a little slower and have to train a little longer, but for those who remain active in their later years, the quality of their life improves.

Sports Medicine Research—Some encouraging scientific reports were presented to the American College of Sports Medicine in 1980. The book *Exercise and Aging* was compiled from these well-documented papers.

Some studies on exercise among those over 65 dealt with cardiovascular benefits, range-of-joint motion, and bone changes.

In his report, Dr. Kenneth H. Sidney observes, "The extent of physiological improvement with endurance training is affected by personal factors such as motivation, attitude and initial health and fitness status, and by program factors such as the type of exercise employed and its duration, frequency and intensity." The first and foremost effect of such regular endurance training is to improve and maintain the oxygen-transport capacity of the cardiovascular system and the *oxidative* capacity of the skeletal muscle groups.

Kathleen Munns researched *range-of-joint motion,* or flexibility, while working on her Ph.D. in exercise physiology. Her study, designed to test the effects of an exercise and dance program, involved volunteers from age 65 to 88. She knew that impaired movement, one of the most pronounced changes associated with advanced age, can result from balance difficulty, loss of muscle strength, and decreased flexibility. In the elderly volunteers who took part in her 12-week study, range-of-joint motion improved significantly.

Bone-mineral decline, called *osteoporosis,* is the primary cause of hip fractures increasing some 50-fold in people between the ages of 40 and 70. It is thought that inactivity might be a cause.

Luckily, bone adapts, like other body tissue. When stressed, it *hypertrophies,* or increases. When unstressed, it atrophies. The growth of bone is dependent to some extent on the amount of stress and strain exerted on it.

In osteoporosis investigations at the University of Wisconsin, Dr. Everett L. Smith, director of the Biogerentology Laboratory, found that when stress and strain is placed on living bone tissue, the physical activity stimulates bone-mineral accumulation—in both young and old.

"Older" Athletes—The athletes in the Masters Division—age 40 and up—whom I have met are dynamic. They don't seem to worry about getting older. In fact, they often welcome birthdays, especially if it puts them in an older age category!

For example, Fred Ellis was highlighted on ABC-TV's coverage of the 1983 Ironman race. Fred, who decided to train for the Ironman after he was treated for cancer, was asked about the possibility of a recurrence. "If it comes back," he said, "it will have to catch me on the move. I'm going to live life to the fullest."

MY PHILOSOPHY FOR YOU

Due to fate and circumstance, I was once a middle-aged woman, no longer needed for the roles for which I'd been raised. I was frightened, insecure and unwilling to reach past the boundaries of house and motherhood. Then I acquired the mindset of an athlete—by the very unscientific method of trial and error. Out of those years of increasing competition, of becoming stronger physically and tougher mentally, the "Millie Brown Fitness Philosophy" evolved.

My philosophy now says: Whatever exercise you do, it should be fun; it should have variety; and it should be free of rigid time schedules. It wasn't prestige that motivated me. I was seeking contentment, health and a new lifestyle, and an escape from tension, anxieties and insecurities. *And I had the rest of my life to do it.*

This Book's Program—The low-stress program of this book embraces this philosophy. It will offer you variety while you achieve a complete workout. It includes instructions on the basics of each type of workout—stretching, walking, bicycling and swimming—and discusses the physiological and psychological benefits. Charts and photos throughout this book will aid you in structuring your program and sticking to it.

It is not necessary to use all of the workouts of this book in your program, although stretching should always be an integral part. You can choose one of the other three, all of them, mix and match, or go from one to another.

I want you to start right now by finishing this book and using its ideas. Don't think of yourself as getting older or being out of shape any longer. Whatever your age, your physical condition or your mental outlook, you *can* better yourself. You *can* rid yourself of negative thoughts, replacing them with positive images and a better body. You must not be afraid to dream. That's a problem with becoming an adult. Too many of us stop imagining ourselves as winners. Find the courage to dream a little, and I will show you how to gain your fitness goals. *You do have the rest of your life!*

CHAPTER TWO

Seven Golden Rules Of Fitness

I have devised a seven-point list of rules or guidelines to lead you through years of enjoyable self-improvement. I think it's important to review and understand these rules before actually starting the low-stress fitness program. They'll give you a better insight into what I'll be asking of you and will supply you with a solid base for devising your own exercise regimen.

The rules are:
1) Positive thoughts only.
2) Dreams into goals.
3) Realistic time schedules.
4) Gather aerobic benefits.
5) Better diet.
6) Listen to your body.
7) Controlling moods.

1) POSITIVE THOUGHTS ONLY

Don't let your exercise program become a self-defeating drudgery or chore. Enough things in our lives get that way as it is, eroding positive images of ourselves. Most people who exercise regularly aren't doing it just because it's good for them. Rather, they do it because it makes them feel good. They have learned that regular exercise is essential to well-being.

I have several friends I see every few months. Rather than visit on the phone or over drinks, we go for long walks or bike rides. Not only are we enjoying each other's company, we're also taking pleasure in nature. We bicycle to a park, walk through the woods and catch up on events in each other's lives. This can be especially therapeutic if one of us is feeling down. Talking things out while exercising your body is a great way to perk up your spirits.

The Rule In Action—When a person is feeling down or depressed, thoughts are dominated by negative feelings. Imperfections and mistakes seem to outweigh all favorable qualities.

My rule is always to think positive thoughts while exercising. I keep a list of some compliments I've received and refer to it when I'm getting depressed. Since I tend to magnify my faults, I focus on praise I've received. As I'm exercising, rather than allow myself to dwell on what I'm not, I think about what I have become.

Generally, people tend to receive more criticism than compliments. Therefore, we need to remember the good. I recommend that you too start a compliment list as a self-pride booster, so you will have concrete proof that you're not so bad.

Here's an example of my chart and a blank one following for you to photocopy. Use it to make your own:

SELF-PRIDE BOOSTER
(I'm Not So Bad After All)

Date	Source	Compliment
8/3/85	Son Mark	"Mom, you change your bike tires like a pro now."
9/5/85	Stranger	"You look so healthy, it must be exercise."
9/12/85	Neighbor	"The garden looks nice now that it's weeded."
9/13/85	Triathlete	"I got into this sport because of you."
9/15/85	Male Friend	"You're looking super! Lost some weight, didn't you?"

SELF-PRIDE BOOSTER
(I'm Not So Bad After All)

Date	Source	Compliment

A Good Addiction—Your goal should be to make your exercise program a "positive addiction." Dr. William Glasser, psychiatrist at the Institute for Reality Therapy in West Los Angeles and author of *Positive Addiction,* suggests anyone can do it as long as he or she follows these guidelines:

1) The activity must be non-competitive and voluntarily selected.

2) It should be something you can do easily and without much mental effort for at least an hour a day.

3) The activity should be one you can do alone and does not depend on the participation of others.

4) The activity must have some physical, emotional or spiritual value for you.

5) You must believe that persistence will result in improvement.

6) Finally, the activity must be one you can do without self-criticism.

Get a Fitness Buddy—Millions of Americans have joined the exercise revolution during the last several years. Half of them drop out. Research indicates the initial six-month period of an exercise program is the critical period. The key is to start a program that is enjoyable and non-stressful—something to look forward to.

As mentioned a bit earlier, one of the best ways to persist is to find a companion to share some of your exercise. Select someone who is compatible with your goals and schedules. If you are sedentary, don't choose someone who is in shape and active. If you're 50 and non-competitive, don't choose a 20-year-old racer.

It's great if you can persuade your mate or a family member to join you. Don't be discouraged, though, if you can't think of anyone. Take the initiative and find a companion. Ask your neighbors, club members or co-workers. Or, take out a short-term membership in an exercise studio and pass the word around that you're looking for companions to join you on walks or bike rides. There are a lot of people we come in contact with who want or need to exercise regularly but need someone to help motivate them.

On the other hand, you may be a person who is surrounded by many people on the job and at home. You need a reprieve from the sound of voices and phones. For you, it might be best to take a walk alone in the park or woods and listen to the sounds of nature. Sometimes, just the sound of your own footsteps can act as a tranquilizer. A swim is another great way to block out annoying sights, sounds and pressures.

Determine which way is best for you—working out alone or in a crowd—and start moving! You can find a million reasons not to get on the bike or in the water.

I find that the best way for *me* to continue my training is to team up with friends.

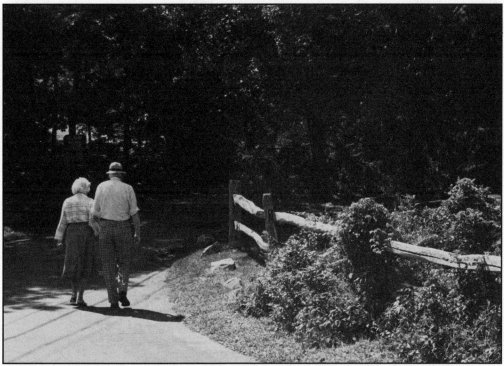
These two walkers are equally fit, so they make perfect fitness buddies.

My friend, Maureen Granito, recently called me on the phone to complain that her training has gone down the drain since I hibernated to finish this book. We had trained together for 18 months after our first meeting. She was training for her first triathlon and was worried about the event. I suggested we do some training, and after some prodding from her husband she gave me a call. Since then we have served as each other's coach and prime motivator. Maureen, who works part time as a nurse, is the mother of four children and hopes to try an Ironman event in a few years.

In the meantime we are starting an exercise group to help others and maintain our own training. Very few people have the discipline to stay with an exercise routine without some commitment, or someone to "egg them on." Maureen and I use the most beautiful facility in the world to workout in with our group—The Great Outdoors.

Natalie Tickner, one of my best friends, has made a resolution to preserve her daily "playtime." She is a vivacious 52-year-old who looks 35. Natalie became a runner and marathoner at the age of 45 after a mastectomy. Several times in her life she let herself become submerged in family problems. Within those periods she was afflicted with hypertension and cancer. She is convinced that her playtime—or exercise time—is a preventive measure against ill health. "If my attitude had been better at those times, I might not have suffered those illnesses." She thinks that cancer and hypertension are partially stress-related, and her playtime gives her relaxation and freedom from stress. "That's my time. It's the one thing I do for myself alone," says Natalie.

Her husband proudly shows off Natalie's running trophies. She has at least 30. "I never won a thing as a kid, and now it's a lot more fun being older."

Learn to Say "I'll try!"—We should ignore all the negative things we fear and feel about ourselves and exercising. Think positively and you can tailor-make your own personal exercise program to be non-stressful, safe and enjoyable. Try to eliminate the phrase, "I can't!" from your vocabulary. Instead say, "I'll try!"

My favorite line after I completed my first Ironman was, "I'll try!" Not only was I saying it, I was doing it, trying things that I had assumed were impossible for me a year before.

"I'll try!" is what I said when Sam Elpern, an ultramarathoner in my running club, suggested I join him in a 12-hour run and also a 50-mile race. (Sam decided to take up running in his late 40s while recovering from double-bypass heart surgery.) I covered 50 miles in the 12-hour race in Prospect Park, New York, learned a lot about what I did wrong, and vowed never to do a crazy thing like that again. I refer to that event as my "pain training."

A month later I was at the start of the 50-mile race at Lake Waramang in Connecticut. I had absolutely no intention of trying to do that distance. I simply wanted to run a few miles around the beautiful lake and meet other racers. My promise to myself was that I would quit at the first sign of pain. I met and ran with Bev Nolan, a 50-year-old secretary who had started endurance runs a few years before. She told me how she completed two *six-day* races within two months, running 50 miles each day. We chatted for 10 miles, then, still feeling relaxed, I took off on my own to enjoy the scenery and some solitude.

It wasn't until 40 miles elapsed that I started to tire. I finished the 50 miles in 9 hours, 30 minutes, felt fine and had no bad after-affects. That convinced me that the secret is to relax and keep free of pressures. We can sometimes do incredible feats under those circumstances.

I also want you to learn from my mistakes. By reading this you should also learn what *not* to try. I learned a lot of things the hard way because there was no one available who had done what I wanted to do. There were a lot of athletes, but it seemed they all had better training and were more dedicated and intense. I'm not one of the best athletes. I'm just an ordinary woman willing to try—one who has taken the words "I can't!" out of her vocabulary.

Many people probably feel as I sometimes did—incapable, inadequate, unworthy and afraid. I hope you can understand me and my effort and that I can inspire you—not necessarily to do ultramarathons or Ironman events—but to make exercise a valuable part of your day.

2) DREAMS INTO GOALS

If you can perceive it, you can achieve it. If you want to lose weight, acquire the radiant look of good health, be in shape, have energy, vitality and endurance, picture yourself that way. Use imagery. Mentally call up images to get yourself "psyched" for your exercise goals.

Spend time each day seeing yourself as you would ideally like to be. That time could be when you first wake up and are still lying in bed, or when you are getting dressed. Look in the mirror, but don't be discouraged at how you may think you look. Instead, visualize looking at the athletic, energetic mind and body that will be yours.

Do some role-playing in your head. Imagine an enjoyable exercise regimen, your involvement in it and the outcome. The idea is to practice new behavior patterns so that when it comes time to actually perform, it will be easy to do.

After a particularly stressful time, or in the evening after a tiring day, sit down for a few minutes, close your eyes, breathe deeply, relax. Know that as you stick with your exercise goals, you will be rewarded with increased energy and more constructive ways of handling stress and anxiety. This can be a quick psychological pick-up.

Dr. Hans Selye, author of *Stress Without Distress,* says this about activity and motivation:

"Activity is a biological necessity. We have seen that unused muscles, brains and organs lose efficiency. To keep fit, we must exercise both our bodies and our minds. Inactivity deprives us of every outlet for our innate urge to create, to build; this causes tensions and the insecurity that stems from aimlessness. Whether we call our activity exhausting work or relaxing play depends largely upon our own attitude towards it.

"Diversion from one activity to another is more relaxing than complete rest. Few things are as frustrating as complete inactivity, the absence of any stimulus, any challenge.

"Deprivation of motivation is the greatest mental tragedy because it destroys all guidelines.

"Motivation, preferably an ambition to accomplish something that really satisfies you and hurts no one, is essential."

Set Goals—Attitude will make or break your fitness program. People who live abundantly have etched an ongoing sense of direction and purpose in their lives. Basic psychology points out the need for goals because they give us reasons for being and doing.

A well-planned system of goals and objectives gives continuity to what we do. We have to decide what we want and acquire a sense of direction. Otherwise, we will end up in circles. We need something to aim for and set our sights on—specific, meaningful goals.

There are always risks involved in setting goals, such as the possibility of not reaching them. Remember, as long as you give an honest and sincere effort, you will not be a failure. If you don't achieve the hoped-for outcome, it may be because you set unrealistic goals or have not put in enough time and effort. I found that it was important to build my confidence slowly, without placing too much pressure on myself at any one time.

Those who lack the courage to live life to the fullest are missing out. Negative people who criticize, condemn and constantly point out others' mistakes are the real failures. We all have met or know those types and what a chore it is to be around them.

Dr. Selye says, "Man must work. We have to begin by clearly realizing that work is a biological necessity. Just as our muscles become flabby and degenerate if not used, so our brain steps into chaos and confusion unless we constantly use it for some work that seems worthwhile to us."

George Bernard Shaw had some thoughts on the subject of work. He said, "Labor is doing what we must; leisure is doing what we like." And, "A perpetual holiday is a good working definition of hell."

Zest for life, enthusiasm, vitality, energy and endurance are within everyone's reach. We need to move our bodies, minds and spirits to keep from becoming stagnant, listless, stale and apathetic. Athletes, artists, inventors and people of vision daydream and, characteristically, are vivacious, spirited and enthusiastic. This is because they are exercising their minds *and* bodies.

Setting goals is a way of making a commitment to optimism. You are taking steps to enrich your future. If you refuse to think about achieving a goal, the odds of obtaining much are slim.

How To Do It—Let's assume that your goals are to lose weight, to firm and tone your body, to improve your cardiovascular system, to increase flexibility, and to acquire more self-confidence and esteem. It's important to clearly identify what you want. This way, it becomes more official and is not easily forgotten.

Writing down goals increases your personal commitment to them. The more details, the more direction you get. Instead of saying, "I am going to lose weight," be specific. Determine the number of pounds you want to lose. Set a realistic time plan. Rapid weight loss and fad diets are not healthy. The diet section in this book has specific tips on losing weight permanently.

You can record cardiovascular improvements by measuring blood pressure and pulse before you start the program. After months of exercise and a low-salt, low-fat diet, a drop in blood pressure will be apparent.

Bend over and see if you can touch your toes without straining. You may only be able to reach your knees. If you stretch consistently and slowly for a few months, you should find yourself touching the floor without effort. Confidence and esteem may be difficult to acquire, but I guarantee that you'll feel confidence returning when you start reaching your daily, weekly and short-term goals.

Be specific about what you must do to achieve your goals. Decide goals for a week, one month and three months. These can be your short- and medium-term goals. Things you want to achieve in half a year up to five years can be long-range and ultimate goals, as shown in some examples that follow.

Make similar forms to determine what your goals are. Set specific short-, medium-, long-range and ultimate goals. Decide how to find the time to fit exercise into your lifestyle and not burn out.

Many of us change with the seasons. Our exercise program may have to change also if we exercise outdoors and live in areas with extreme weather changes.

We also change with age as we grow and enter into different life stages. Psychological research has shown that adults face different challenges and crisis periods every five to eight years. With that in mind, keep your long-term goals

SHORT-TERM GOALS
FOR THE WEEK

DIET

OBJECTIVE:	Lose one pound.
MOTIVATION:	My skirt not pinching my waist.
EFFORT:	Cut down on salt.
REWARD:	One red rose.

EXERCISE

OBJECTIVE:	Not to feel tired at 7 p.m.
MOTIVATION:	Arrange to exercise with a friend.
EFFORT:	Exercise from 5:30 to 6:30.
REWARD:	Glass of my favorite white wine.

SELF-ESTEEM

OBJECTIVE:	Be less selfish.
MOTIVATION:	Read an inspiring story.
EFFORT:	Take my blind friend ice skating.
REWARD:	Enjoy my blind friend's gratitude.

MEDIUM-TERM GOALS

IN 1 MONTH
Lose two pounds.
Meet a new friend to exercise with.
Stop telling myself I look fat.

IN 3 MONTHS
Lose two more pounds.
Cut salt consumption.

IN 6 MONTHS
Cut alcoholic consumption in half.
Exercise five times per week.
Feel proud of myself.

IN 9 MONTHS
Have more energy and stamina.
Feel athletic.
Cut fat and sugar consumption.

LONG-TERM GOALS

IN 1 YEAR
Exercise will be a positive addiction.
Major reduction in fats, salts, sugar and alcohol from diet.
Fit into smaller-size clothes.
Stop smoking.

IN 2-1/2 YEARS
Enter an athletic event that would have been impossible three years ago.
Do not regain lost weight.
No longer have desire for foods that aren't healthy.

IN 5 YEARS
Aging is not a concern because I'm improving.
I have gained self-confidence by knowing I can achieve realistic goals.

within a five-year period. It helps to set a five-year long-range goal, as that alleviates the pressure of trying to do something too fast.

For example, my own needs have changed since I've turned 45. My "mid-life crisis" has passed and I no longer feel that I have to prove anything to myself or others. My goals are changing from the need to strive and compete to that of wanting to help others achieve health and happiness.

3) REALISTIC TIME SCHEDULES

You may think that finding the time to exercise is an insurmountable problem. Actually you just need to be creative. There is a lot of truth in the saying, "If you want something done, ask a busy person."

When I was training for triathlons, I was working and attending college, so I combined social activities with training. In addition, a lot of studying was accomplished on long, slow solitary runs. A small tape recorder enabled me to review class lectures and notes. Many term papers were composed while I was moving.

Studies have shown (and I can personally attest to the fact) that people become more creative when involved in aerobic activities—those that work your heart and lungs steadily. During aerobic exercise, our brains are being supplied with more oxygen. A good investment for business people would be a micro-cassette recorder they could take when walking or cycling. They could record ideas or solutions to problems that pop into their heads while in the relaxed state of rhythmic exercise.

A stationary bicycle is another good way of fitting exercise into a busy lifestyle. You can watch the TV news or your favorite program while working out on the bike.

If your life is demanding, it will benefit you in the long run to put aside one hour a day for yourself. Break it up into three 20-minute exercise breaks if you find it impossible to fit in one hour at a stretch. Mothers with family responsibilities and people with job obligations get so caught up in the pressures of constantly doing things for others that they think they have no time for themselves. I remember how frustrating it was for me before I started exercising regularly. When I started giving myself at least one hour a day to walk or run away from my pressures or obligations, I stopped feeling like a martyr. Make it a hard-and-fast rule to take that hour a day for yourself.

Find the Motivation—There is no one fitness program that is best. It must be tailor-made to your personality and lifestyle. Only you can determine what your motivating factors are. Perhaps you are motivated by desire for career promotion or change. Improved health and increased stamina are definite advantages. Or, you may yearn for a more attractive outward appearance. Proper diet and exercise can contribute to a natural, glowing beauty.

Would the prospect of a more exciting life motivate you? The energy and self-confidence produced through exercise *can* enable you to find that. Would you like to be able to cope better with stress and anxiety? An aerobic exercise program will help you cope.

Morning Exercise—If you're a "morning person," it would probably be best to schedule your exercise time in the morning. You may have to get up earlier, but your body will soon adjust, and the rewards will be worth it.

Warning: Morning exercisers need a longer warm up time. A study of runners in California showed a higher percentage of running-related injuries such as pulled muscles and tendonitis in morning runners. It has also been suggested that temperature is a major contributing factor to the higher injury rate for those who run in the morning.

Humans are subjected to *circadian rhythms*—biological clocks—that control everything from mental performance to emotional stability. These rhythms also control our body temperature, which peaks during the middle of the day and falls to its lowest point during the early morning hours. Between 4 and 6 a.m. the body is the coolest, and body processes—called *metabolism*—are at their lowest levels.

Shortly after waking, your body is often at a "subnormal" state. The chance of stress-induced injury is magnified by the shock your body receives in going from rest to vigorous exercise. After you have been in bed resting all night, soft tissues contract. That's why you need the longer warmup in the morning.

In my low-stress fitness program, you give yourself adequate time to enjoy the walk, the stretches, the morning bike ride or swim. People who once hated the idea of being an early riser find early mornings the most peaceful time of the day. I absolutely love the freshness of the morning and the splendor of a sunrise! Morning exercise can be more addictive, according to some studies, possibly because it's easier to fit exercise into a busy schedule the first thing in the morning.

A lack of energy in the morning could be caused by a short supply of stored "sugars" in the liver. The liver can store only enough of this substance—called *glycogen*—to last 12 hours at rest, according to Dr. Gabe Mirkin. The brain derives about 98% of its energy from blood sugar. You have only enough sugar in your bloodstream to last about three minutes.

So to keep your blood sugar level up, the liver constantly releases sugar into the bloodstream. As you exercise, you may develop a low blood-sugar level and feel weak because your muscles and brain aren't getting enough fuel.

To avoid this, drink a glass of orange juice or eat a piece of toast right before you exercise to get an immediate energy boost. If you eat a large meal, wait an hour before exercising.

Midday Exercise—Noon also is a good time to fit in a brisk walk. It will improve afternoon productivity and is a good way to relieve morning stress.

Evening Exercise—"Evening people" balk at the idea of exercising in the morning. For them to introduce a new activity at a time of the day when they feel low can be defeating. And there is a lot to be said for exercising later in the day. A stressful day can lead to the production and accumulation of adrenal fluids. Exercise lets our bodies remove this "stress," allowing us to return to a more relaxed state. Having a cocktail or reading the paper after a tough day *will not* relieve your tensions as effectively as exercise.

Research at Dr. Cooper's Aerobics Center suggests that the timing of your exercise may have an effect on the control of fat and weight. Dr. Cooper recommends that you engage in aerobic exercise prior to a meal and preferably the evening meal. "If you exercise no earlier than two hours prior to the meal you'll be more likely to lose a larger percent of body fat than if you exercise at other times of the day. It is also known that the body metabolism tends to increase during the day and then slow down as nighttime approaches," he says. "As a result, you tend to burn less calories in the evening than earlier in the day. If you exercise late in the afternoon, you may be increasing the pace of your metabolism and simultaneously increasing the ability of your body to burn more calories in the evening."

Strategy—If you know your biological clock and your peak time of the day, go with it. Until we have proven to ourselves how much better we feel by being fit and have formed a positive addiction, we need to do everything we can to stay on course. Basically, you should exercise just before you want to be most alert. Exercise increases your temperature and your mental alertness for four to six hours. Because of this you may have some trouble sleeping if you exercise too close to bedtime.

To help decide what hours you can set aside for your fitness program, get a wall calendar and put down all the things you regularly do—job, shopping, children—and circle those times you can steal for yourself. As I said, an hour at a time is best, but if that can't be done, then work on three 20-minute segments.

Once you have selected these exercise times, mark them so they stand out. Mark each week this way for the entire month. At the beginning of a new month, start all over again. Hang the calendar where you can't help but see it.

Self-Discipline—Keep in mind that staying with an exercise routine will not only improve you physically, but can make you a more disciplined person in other areas. When you acquire more self-discipline, you'll have the strength to make changes in your habits. Then you will see positive personality changes.

You develop courage by tackling something beneficial and staying with it. Someone remarked to me how courageous I was to finish the Ironman. My reply was, "The real courage was in mailing in my application."

I have cultivated the ability to follow through and finish tasks that previously I'd leave uncompleted. If I start a race, I finish it, no matter how long I take. I quit only for medical reasons, not if I tire. I have taught myself to make the best of things. Even in my worst Ironman (1983), in which I had a lot of difficulty and finished four minutes before the race cutoff, I was able to joke with the cameramen following me. Consequently, I've developed a stick-to-itiveness in other areas of my life.

Make it Easy—Select a convenient location to keep your exercise gear—bike by the back door, walking shoes in the front of your closet, swimming gear all in one spot. In other words, do all you can before you exercise to make it easier for you to go out and actually do it.

It's important to take part in a variety of exercises, in different settings. Your goal is to exercise different groups of muscles. Combining walking, bicycling, swimming and stretching does this admirably. My low-stress fitness program ensures a full-body workout, following the hard/easy method of training.

Change and variety will help keep you motivated, enthusiastic, and not let exercise become a negative addiction—unenjoyable and domineering.

I've seen real obsession among runners and triathletes and have been guilty of it myself at times. I suppose it also occurs with tennis, skiing and other sports. If you tend to be a compulsive type, seek a better balance. One hour a day devoted to moderate exercise will do this.

Aerobic activities, aside from improving your cardiovascular system, offer emotional and character-building benefits. I can attest to the fact that researchers postulate: The hypnotically repetitive rhythm of aerobic sports causes positive alterations in thought, resulting in increased self-assurance, esteem, perseverance, determination and courage.

Perseverance, endurance and tenacity are the fringe benefits of sticking with something until you reach a goal. Raising children or remaining with a boring job may have already given you those traits. Now use them in your low-stress fitness program.

The basic message in the third rule is to not expect too much too soon. Be realistic. Dramatic changes will not occur overnight. Give yourself plenty of time. If you set your beginning goals too high and try to achieve them too quickly, you will become discouraged and drop out.

4) GATHER AEROBIC BENEFITS

Aerobic exercises require steady, above-normal cardiovascular and respiratory action for a certain minimum time. This stimulates the need for large quantities of oxygen. Ultimately, this forces the body to improve the systems responsible for oxygen transport. For example, walking, swimming, bicycling, jogging, running, skating, rowing, and cross-country skiing, among others, are

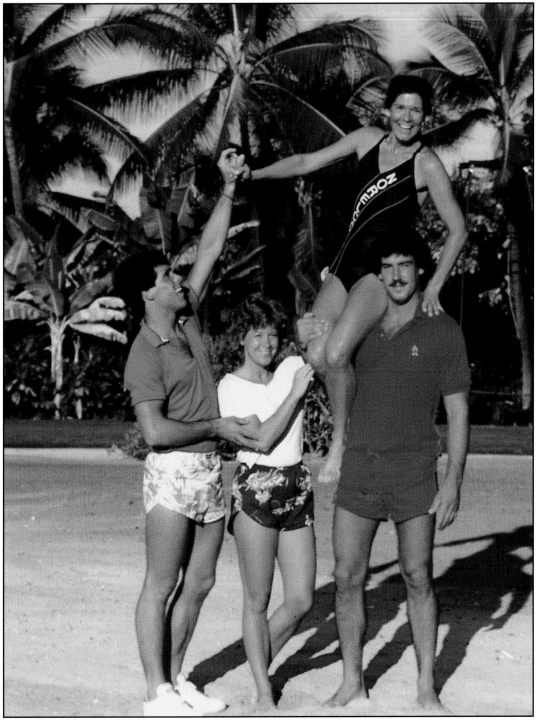

Getting in shape is easier and more satisfying if you get support from family and friends. My "strongest" supporters are my three children—left to right, Mark, Chris and Larry. Photo by Bill Travis.

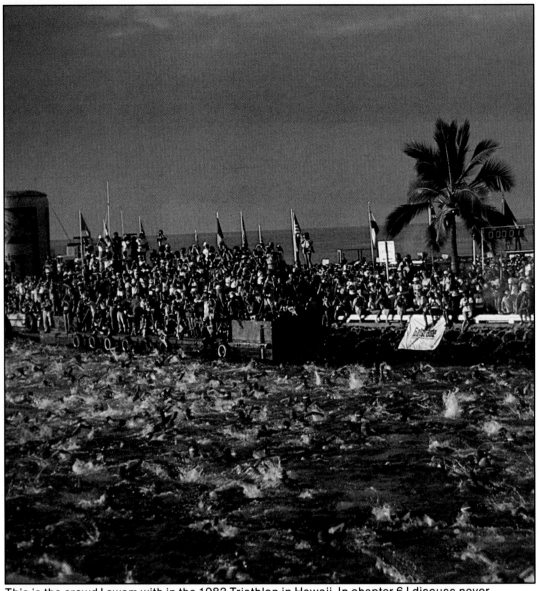

This is the crowd I swam with in the 1983 Triathlon in Hawaii. In chapter 6 I discuss never swimming alone, but don't suggest that you need to go to this extreme!

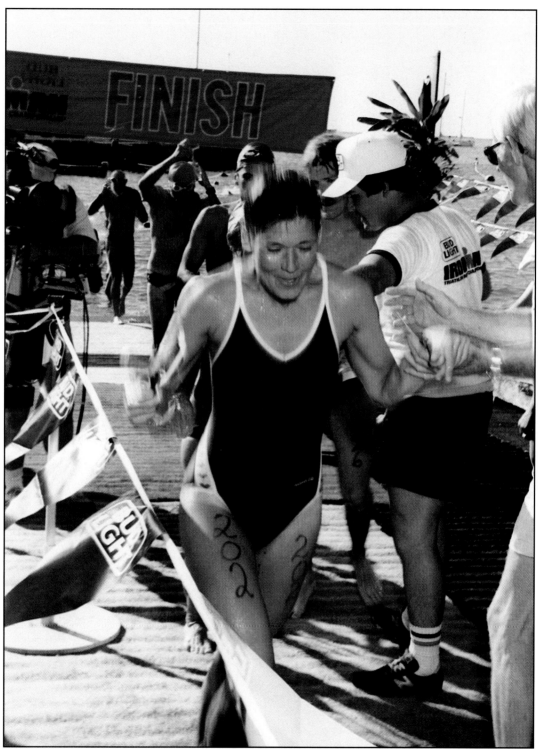

Here, I've just finished the 2.4 mile swim in the 1983 Hawaii Triathlon.

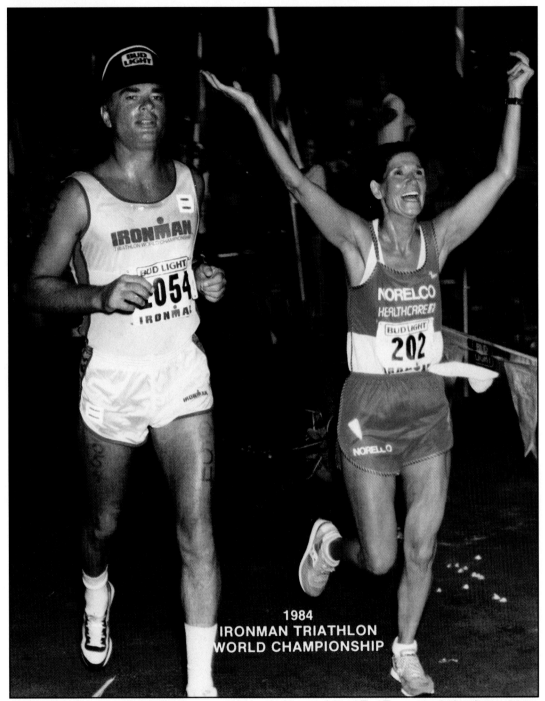

1984
IRONMAN TRIATHLON
WORLD CHAMPIONSHIP

At the 1984 Triathlon finish line I was accompanied by my friend Ted Treu, who helped me throughout the event. Whether you compete or exercise for fun, you will benefit from a fitness buddy.

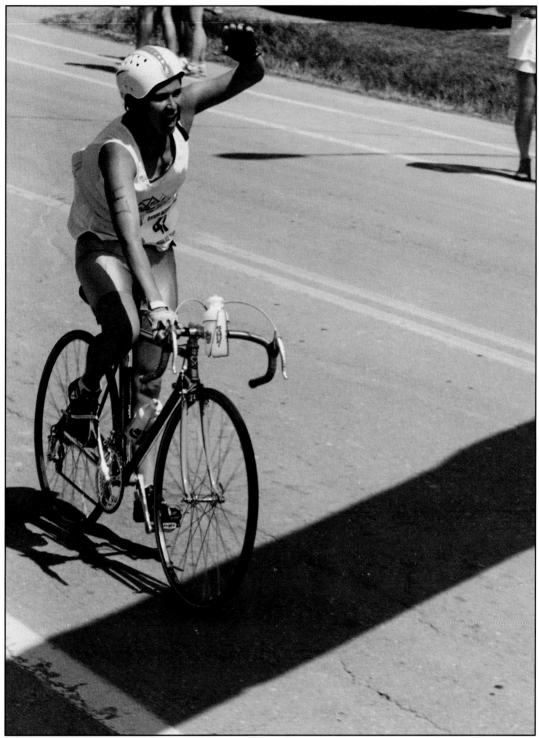

I don't expect to win every competition I enter. The thrill of participation usually supplies enough satisfaction for me. That's why in chapter 7 I suggest you try some fun competitions.

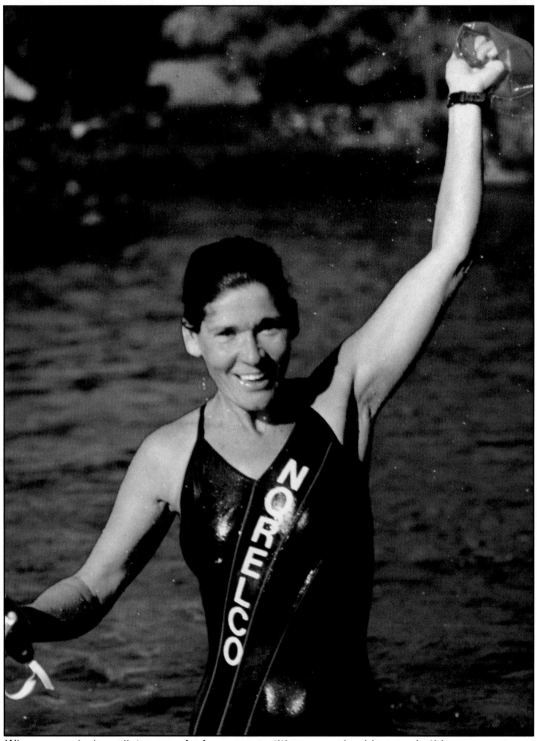

When you swim long distances—for fun or competition—you should wear a bathing cap, goggles and a tight-fitting swimsuit. Photo by Bill Travis.

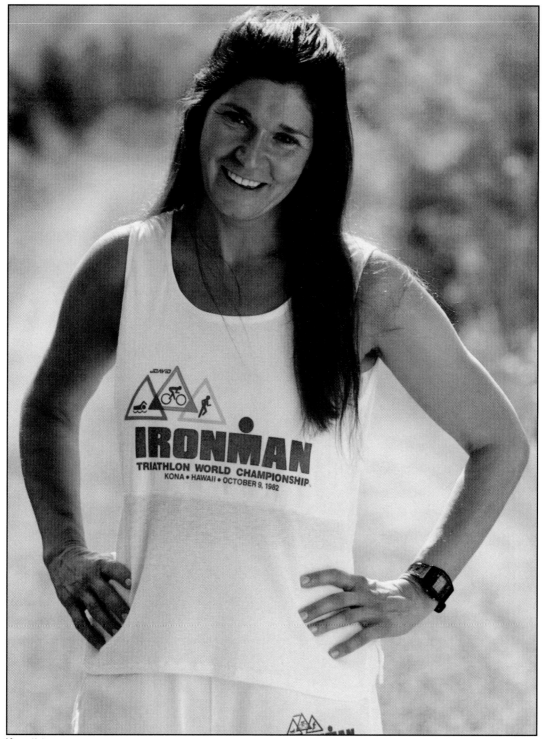

If walking and running long distances, you'll enjoy yourself more in sports clothing. I wear special shirts and shorts to avoid chafing and other discomfort. Photo by Barbara Walz.

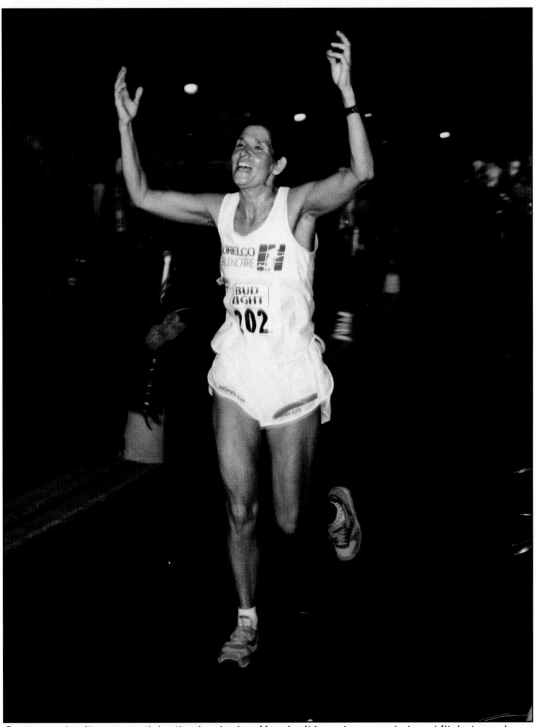

On the road to fitness, participating is winning. You don't have to compete to get fit, but you do have to "enter the event." The best part about low-stress fitness is that you have the rest of your life to achieve your goals.

considered aerobic *if* you do them steadily at a rhythmic pace.

When judging an activity for its aerobic benefits, use the following criteria:

1) Large muscle groups should be used.

2) Do the activity a minimum of three days per week, preferably on alternate days.

3) The activity should be maintained continuously, at low intensity, for 20 to 45 minutes and should be rhythmical in nature.

4) During this time, you should work to bring your heart rate up to your *target heart rate* (THR), described a bit later.

5) Warm up before and cool down afterward by walking slowly. You should not stop suddenly after vigorous exercise.

Determining Target Heart Rate—This heart rate is a measure of the minimal intensity of exercise that will condition muscles and the cardiovascular system. The end result is physical fitness. The target heart rate is not overly strenuous. In fact, on average it is from 70% to 85% of your maximum aerobic ability.

To determine your approximate target heart rate, use the following formulas:

$$220 - \text{Your Age} = \text{Maximum Heart Rate (MHR)}$$
$$\text{MHR} \times (70\% \text{ to } 85\%) = \text{Target Heart Rate (THR)}$$

For example, a 45-year-old woman has a maximum heart rate (MHR) of $220 - 45 = 175$. If she does not exercise regularly, her target heart rate (THR) should be about $175 \times .70 = 119$. If she is in excellent physical condition, her target heart rate is about $175 \times .85 = 149$.

To measure your heart rate, learn to count your pulse at the wrist on the thumb side with your opposite index finger. Or, place an index finger on the carotid artery under your jaw. Count your pulse immediately upon stopping the activity because the rate changes very quickly once you slow down or stop. Find the beat within a second, then count for 6 seconds. Multiply this number by 10 to obtain your heart rate (HR) per minute.

For example, if you count 13 beats in 6 seconds, your heart rate per minute is 130. If you are 45 years old and could keep up that heart rate for 20 minutes minimum, I'd say that you are in fine aerobic shape.

What Will Happen—Exercising to reach your target heart rate for 20 to 45 minutes will eventually lower blood pressure and resting heart rate. This means that the heart needs less oxygen. When fit, you put less strain on the cardiovascular system. The chances of sustaining a heart attack or having another if you have already been stricken will probably be decreased.

Aerobic exercise also changes the clotting power of the blood, making it less likely to clot in coronary arteries.

Endurance-building exercises, along with a low-fat diet, have been shown

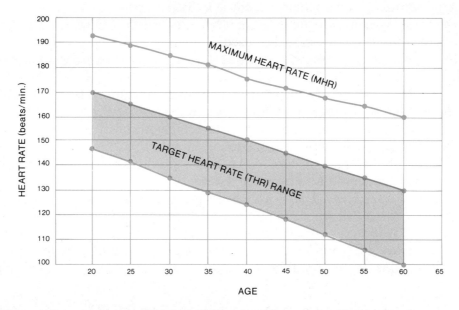

This graph is a summary of the formulas on the previous page. The graph shows that as you get older, your highest attainable heart rate decreases. The formulas and graph results are averaged values, not exact values. They are generally true for most people. It *is* possible for a normal, 50-year-old man to have an MHR of 195 or a 30-year-old man to have an MHR of 168. From *Beyond Diet: Exercise Your Way to Fitness and Heart Health* by Lenore R. Zohman, M. D.

to reduce blood cholesterol and body weight. The way the body handles carbohydrates is improved, and there is less "adrenalin-type" chemical secreted by the body in response to emotional stress than in unfit people.

Another great benefit of aerobic exercise is that it's one of the best ways to "convert" fat to muscle. A lot of the standard weight charts are obsolete or misleading. Scales can be very deceiving because they show only total weight. I have felt fat and bloated at times and lean and slender at other times—even though my weight was about the same.

I was part of a research project at the University of Pennsylvania. Dr. Douglas Hiller, a research associate at Penn's Institute for Environmental Medicine and an Ironman himself, tested a group of Ironmen and Ironwomen. We went through a battery of medical tests, several of them to assess our body composition.

I accompanied Eva Ueltzen, third place in the 1983 Ironman, to the underwater weighing laboratory. We were weighed on a scale before being submerged in the tank to determine how much of our body weight was fat. I was amazed to find out how much Eva, a 27-year-old triathlete, weighed. But tests showed that she had proportionately more muscle than fat.

The standard age-height-weight charts reveal little about an individual's body composition. It is possible to be overweight and not overfat. This is the case in some athletes, especially football players.

About Fat—Total body fat exists in two states—*essential* and *storage*. Essential fat is stored in the marrow of bones and in the heart, lungs, liver, spleen, kidneys, intestines, muscles, and lipidrich tissues throughout the central nervous system. The fat is required for normal physiological functioning. In women, essential fat also includes sex-specific, or sex-characteristic, fat. The breasts and the pelvic region are primary storage sites for this fat.

The other major fat, storage fat, consists of fat accumulated in adipose tissue. This nutritional reserve includes the fatty tissue that protects various internal organs from trauma, as well as the larger subcutaneous fat deposited beneath the skin.

Many people carry anywhere from 5 to 50 pounds of excess fat in adipose tissue. Try carrying around a 5-pound bag of potatoes or a 20-pound load and see how quickly you tire. Think how much more energy you could have and how much better you would feel if you weren't lugging around extra fat.

True sex differences exist for quantities of essential fat. The average storage fat value for men is 12% of body weight; for women about 15% of body weight. But the essential fat differences are large—men average 3% of body weight, and women about 12% of body weight. The difference is probably related to childbearing and hormonal functions.

Statistics and trends show that with increasing age, body fat increases in both sexes, probably because of inactivity. Cutting down the level of daily physical activity can cause a relative increase in body fat. This occurs even if the daily caloric consumption remains constant. Studies also show that participation in vigorous physical activities after age 35 can retard the average increases in body fat.

What has become an average weight for Americans is not necessarily good. Our goal in achieving and maintaining an athletic body-fat weight should be around 15% to 19% for men, and 18% to 25% for women.

You can determine your body composition in a couple of ways. *Hydrostatic,* or underwater, weighing is one method, but is unavailable to most people. Another is the prediction method. It uses equations developed from relationships between selected skinfolds or circumference measurements and body density or percentage of fat. You also need a special caliper for measuring the body fat, scientific charts and training in the procedures.

Your Ideal Weight—Dr. Kenneth Cooper has developed a formula for the average person to calculate his or her ideal weight.

Men should take their height in inches, multiply it by 4, and subtract 128. Women should take their height in inches, multiply it by 3.5 and subtract 108. This will determine the ideal body weight for men of medium structure with roughly 15% to 19% body fat, and for women of average build with about 18% or 22% body fat.

The most important thing in a weight-loss program is to lower your percentage of body fat, not just to lose pounds. The wrong kind of diet can actually make you fatter by goofing up your metabolism. The physical activity of aerobic exercise subtly resets the systems that control metabolism, causing you to burn more calories.

About Metabolism—An understanding of metabolism may help you achieve a balance between the number of calories consumed and the number your body needs. The *basal metabolic rate,* or BMR, is the minimum level of energy required to sustain the body's vital functions in the waking state.

Energy metabolism at rest is proportional to body surface area. Resting metabolism is about 5% to 10% lower in women than in men. That is due largely to the fact that women generally possess more body fat than men of similar size. And, fat is metabolically less active than muscle. As we get older, our resting metabolic rate slows down.

Therefore, as you get older, you should need fewer calories to sustain you. Generally, if you consume more calories than you need, you will gain weight. Unfortunately, this concept has been oversimplified by many designers of quick-weight-loss diets. Such diets can be very popular, but research shows some of them backfire when rapidly lost weight is quickly regained. This is called the *yo-yo effect.*

Severe caloric restriction forces the body to respond as if it is starving. It conserves energy by lowering the metabolic pacemaker. If we eat small amounts of food frequently, our systems have a constant energy source. But if we eat only one meal a day, the body cannot tell a strict diet from a famine. So, it converts more food to body fat, or adipose fat cells, as a survival measure. Children recovering from serious malnutrition often regain until they become obese.

This over-compensation was discovered long ago by scientists experimenting with lab rats. One group of rats was deprived of food, then allowed to feed freely. The other group never "dieted." The rats deprived of food earlier quickly regained weight and became heavier than the non-dieting rats.

This over-compensation principle has been used by cattle raisers who underfeed the animals before fattening them, creating a cheap way of increasing fat content just before market. In the human condition, crash dieting sets up a yo-yo pattern of loss and rebound gain.

Dr. Paul Ernsberger did his doctoral thesis on the effects of the yo-yo syndrome on blood pressure. He found that over-compensation is kicked off by a profound dietary shock to the system—perhaps a 20% loss of weight—and is fueled at cellular and hormonal levels.

During a diet, fat cells *shrink*. They never disappear. When normal eating is resumed, the fat cells don't just fill up with fat. They can increase in number, *and* refill. New fat cells are there forever too, and they encourage your body to accumulate more fat. Cutting calories can turn out to be the great fattener. Five-year, follow-up records show a third to half the dieters gained back more weight than they initially lost.

Studies have found that as weight goes down, there is loss in both fat and protein, but the regained weight is largely fat. The way to lose weight for good is through aerobic exercise and proper eating habits. We need a well-balanced diet to maintain proper health. In many fad diets, rapid weight-loss is usually just a loss of water caused by the dieuretic action of recommended foods. The dieters are thrilled and think they are losing fat when it is actually only water.

For long-term weight loss, I recommend aerobic exercise. Walking, swimming and bicycling qualify if you do them as I describe in this book. Fat will burn off and muscle will tone. Avoid crash diets that can cause metabolism to readjust to a reduced caloric level.

5) BETTER DIET

Many of us need to change poor eating habits caused by cultural factors and lack of nutritional information. Most Americans eat a diet high in protein and fats but low in complex carbohydrates. This can increase the incidence of heart disease, diabetes, digestive cancers and other degenerative diseases.

In 1977, the Senate Committee on Nutrition and Human Need redefined the concept of a balanced diet. It recommended, in light of modern nutritional and biochemical research, a diet made up of 15% to 20% protein, 20% to 30% fats and 50% to 65% complex carbohydrates.

Protein—You need it daily to maintain growth, promote normal functioning and repair body tissues. Protein-rich foods include meats, fish, poultry, cheese, milk, eggs, dried peas and beans, peanut butter and yogurt. Try to get your protein from foods low in fats. Choose low-fat milk, cheeses and yogurt. Remember poultry, fish and veal are lower in fats then beef, pork or lamb.

Fats—There are two kinds of food fats, *saturated* and *unsaturated*. Unsaturated fats are liquid at room temperature and come from vegetable sources. Saturated fatty acids are from animal sources and are usually solid at room temperature, such as lard. The majority of our fats should be unsaturated, from vegetable sources.

Carbohydrates—Complex carbohydrates are the most readily available sources of food energy. They are the fuel needed by your brain and nerve cells. They provide vitamins, minerals and fiber and are relatively low in calories. Good sources are fresh fruits and vegetables, potatoes, grains (wheat, oats, corn, rice) and grain products (breads, cereals, pasta). Avoid highly processed foods such as white flour and white rice. The only nutrient category not linked to any debilitating or deadly disease is natural, unrefined carbohydrates.

Salt—Limit your salt (sodium chloride) intake. The average American consumes between 3 to 15 times the amount of salt needed. We need only between one-half and two grams of sodium daily. Excess sodium has been linked with high blood pressure, kidney distress, anxiety, overweight and edema (water-logged tissues). Some researchers even think there is a relationship between excess salt and premenstrual syndrome (PMS).

Fluid retention, which can happen to anyone who consumes too much salt, can cause swelling in the abdomen, breasts, ankles, feet, hands, and even the brain. As brain membranes become swollen with water, headaches and migraines may result. Water retention can also lead to depression. It is thought that changes in water, salt, and potassium levels can lead to chemical changes in the nervous system, possibly producing a depressed mood. Fluid retention may be responsible for emotional changes as well such as tension, mood swings, depression, lethargy, fatigue, anger and anxiety.

Many of us have been brought up on salt-laden foods. Many of the processed baby foods we ate were high in sodium. Parents would be wise to nip the salt habit in the bud by selecting salt-free and low-salt foods for their infants. A child's taste buds are in the formulative stage until the age two or three. If babies are given a wide variety of foods without salt, they will grow up to appreciate the natural flavor of foods.

Here's a good rule of thumb regarding salt or sodium intake: Canned or processed foods are the higher in sodium than fresh, unsalted foods. Read labels. It's not unusual to see several types of sodium compounds on a list of ingredients. The following words all indicate sodium: *salt, baking powder, brine, monosodium glutumate, sodium benzoate, sodium bicarbonate, sodium sulfite, sodium hydroxide, sodium cyclamate, baking soda, sodium algenate, sodium propionate, bicarbonate of soda and sodium (Na).*

It is important to learn about the amounts of sodium in foods and beverages. We can't rely on taste alone. I've compiled some facts and composed some lists of high-sodium foods to help guide you.

Domestic red wine contains twice the amount of sodium as imported. Four ounces of domestic white wine contains 19mg compared with 2mg found in imported wine. Imported mineral water has 42mg sodium in an 8-ounce serving. Beer has more sodium than gin, rum, vodka or whiskey. Club soda contains 39mg sodium.

SODIUM CONTENT OF COMMON FOODS

Food	Amount	Sodium (mg)
Corned beef	3.5 oz.	1740
Beef stroganoff	4 oz.	768
Beef teriyaki	4 oz.	1840
Boullion cube	1 cube	960
Fried chicken	4.5 oz.	865
Chicken (stir-fried)	2 oz.	700
Chicken a la king	1 cup	765
Chicken cacciatore	1 serving	1030
Chicken pot pie, frozen	1	939
Chili con carne	1 cup	1338
Chop suey with meat	1 cup	1389
Crabmeat, canned	3.5 oz.	1000
Frankfurters, beef	1.5 oz.	460
Smoked herring	3 oz.	5234
Meatloaf	4.5 oz.	650
Ham	3.5 oz.	1100
French toast	2 slices	550
Kabobs: beef, peppers, barbecue sauce	5 oz.	680
Lasagne with meat sauce	6-7 ozs.	1330
Macaroni and cheese	1 cup	1094
Manicotti with beef, and cheese	2 shells	870
Pizza, sausage	1 slice	546
Scalloped potatoes w/cheese	1 cup	1103
Potato salad	1 cup	1331
Enriched white rice	1 cup	773
Spaghetti, tomato sauce, cheese	1 cup	963
Tomato juice	1 cup	483
Bran flakes with raisins	1 cup	403
Bread stuffing	1 cup	544
Farina	1 cup	469
Oat cereal, toasted wheat germ	1 cup	706
Oatmeal or rolled oats, cooked	1 cup	527
Enriched wheat flour self-rising	1 cup	1360
Apple pie	1 piece	409
Pretzels	1 oz.	480
Garlic salt	1 tsp.	1850
Gravy	1/3 cup	515
Dill pickle	1 med.	934
Table salt	1 tsp.	1993
Soy sauce	1 tbs.	1318

Commercial fruit juices such as apple, orange, grape, lemonade and grape-fruit contain 2 to 3mg of sodium per cup. Sweetened citrus juices (canned or reconstituted) are higher in sodium than fresh-squeezed. Tomato juice has 483mg of sodium per cup.

Coffee and tea are very low in sodium, but cocoa mix prepared with water contains 232mg for one cup.

The sodium content in milk varies among whole, canned and dry. Compare the following one-cup portions: Whole or low-fat milk has about 150mg sodium. Canned milk has 325mg, dry whole milk has 521mg and dry skim, nonfat milk contains 246mg sodium.

Salt Substitutes—Some food-processing companies are now marketing low-sodium products. I tried them before I broke my salt habit and found them too bland. I finally realized that my taste buds were addicted to salt. It took me two weeks of "cold turkey" for my palate to become acquainted with the delights of unsalted foods and other spices.

A sprinkling of other spices in place of salt can make for lively meals. Lemon is a great salt substitute. I use it on fresh vegetables in place of butter and salt. Avoid adding salt to the water when you cook. Try lemon juice or a piece of lemon peel in the water when cooking pasta. Cooking with wine is also fun and tasty. The alcohol vaporizes, leaving flavors behind.

Onions, green pepper and garlic—raw, cooked, powdered and flaked—are other salt substitutes. Spices such as pepper, curry, oregano and cinnamon can liven up your meals too.

Water—When you think you are hungry and head for the refrigerator or cupboard, tell yourself to wait 10 minutes before eating. In the meantime have a large glass of ice water. Enjoy a steaming cup of herbal tea or a diet soda, preferably caffeine-free and low in sodium.

Hunger is often thirst in disguise, so drink water before eating. In fact, drink at least eight glasses of water daily. I drink some of my water in big frosty mugs, or elegant crystal wine glasses, often laced with a slice of fresh lemon or lime. When at social gatherings or home watching television have a glass of water along with a caloric or alcoholic beverage you may be drinking. Alternate drinking from each glass. It's usually habit that brings the drink to our mouths.

Diet Switches—Learn the caloric content of foods and beverages. Increase low-calorie items and restrict high-calorie items. The difference in calories is saved weight. Basically, you gain a pound of weight when you consume 3,500 extra calories.

Better Eating Habits—Many of our eating habits are a matter of reflex. We eat according to a pattern, enjoying particular foods at the same time of the day, in similar circumstances. Check your food list to verify this. It takes conscious thought to change these patterns. A lot of times you may not even be hungry but have developed unconscious eating habits. You must be aware of them to change them. For permanent weight-control, you must establish good, lifelong eating and exercise habits.

Purchasing the right foods is the first step toward proper eating. Try not to go grocery shopping when you are hungry. Buy natural foods, unprocessed whole grains, fresh fruits and vegetables. Reward yourself with non-food items. Figure out the times of the day you are most vulnerable to poor eating habits. Then schedule a different activity for that time.

Preparing and Eating Foods—Purchase and eat foods that are as fresh as possible. The longer they sit in the refrigerator, the more precious nutrients are lost. Frozen foods are second to fresh in retaining nutrients.

When cooking, the less water you use, the better. Steam vegetables or cook them in a microwave. Skin poultry and trim excess fat from meat. Broil or bake meats on a rack. Avoid fried foods. Steam-fry foods in water, not fat. Oriental stir-frying is number one when it comes to retaining nutrients but can be high in fat and salt because of oil and soy sauce. Cook in iron pots if possible. Food cooked in iron pots may contain three to four times more iron than foods cooked in glass or aluminum pots.

Choose skim milk over whole milk. Limit sauces, butter, mayonnaise and dressings, especially creamy ones. Eat bread, rolls and popcorn without the butter. Take servings one-half to two-thirds the usual. Don't feel compelled to eat everything on your plate. Eat off smaller dishes. Use luncheon plates rather than dinner plates. Use half the amount of jellies and syrup at breakfast. If you like nuts, buy them in the shell. They take longer to eat that way.

Eating a wide variety of good foods increases the probability of ingesting essential nutrients. Meals should include a combination of carbohydrates, protein and fats in the recommended proportions—50% carbohydrates, 20% protein and 30% fats.

I think you should know the amounts of protein, fats, carbohydrates and sodium found in your favorite foods. I recommend a pocket-sized book that contains much of this information. It is called *Eat Smart: The Random House Guide To Diet & Nutrition.*

Eat slowly and enjoy your food. Chew it thoroughly. Don't gulp it down. Instead of three large meals, eat five or six small ones.

It's very important to eat a good breakfast. This is the meal most people scrimp on or skip altogether.

Dr. Kenneth Cooper is convinced that if you consume the largest proportion of your calories before 1 p.m. you will have less of a problem controlling your weight than if you consume the same number of calories after 1 p.m.

A recent study at his Aerobics Center in Dallas, Texas, confirmed this. He recommends that everyone try to skew calorie consumption more heavily in the morning and early afternoon hours. Your body metabolism tends to increase during the day, then slows down as nighttime approaches. As a result, you tend to burn less calories in the evening than earlier in the day.

Vitamin and Mineral Supplements—Whether or not we need vitamin and mineral supplements is still controversial. It seems the more I researched it, the more confused I became. One group claims that if we eat a normal diet, we get all the necessary nutrients. Another group claims that because of pollutants in our environment, food additives, processing, loss of nutrients in transportation and storage—among other reasons—our foods lack what we need for proper nutrition.

Vitamins do not contain calories, so extra vitamins will not provide more energy. There may be a small psychological boost in taking supplements. I've observed this among many of my athletic friends. To be on the safe side I suggest taking a good multiple-vitamin capsule daily, plus a vitamin C tablet.

More than half of all American women don't meet the recommended daily amount for calcium. It is also difficult for a woman to get enough iron in her diet, so women should consider taking an extra iron supplement. To maximize absorption, take such supplements with meals.

My Daily Habit—We all have different tastes, habits and lifestyles to take into consideration in regard to diet. I love food! The idea of eating liquid or powdered meals for all the needed vitamins and minerals leaves me cold. I want the pleasure of seeing the different shapes and colors of my sustenance. The variety of smells, tastes and textures of food excites my palate and increases my enjoyment of meals. I have gained quite a reputation of being a big eater. People I worked with were constantly saying, "Millie, you're always eating, but you stay so thin. How do you do it?"

My secret is extending meals over several hours and being conscious of the food's composition. The accompanying table illustrates a typical daily menu.

Most people would have these meals at three different sittings. Instead I break *each meal* into three snacks. Consequently, I'm eating 10 or 11 times a day. This works great for me since I'm single, my children are grown and I have a job that permits this type of eating pattern.

When I ate with the family, I would eat large meals that could leave me feeling bloated and lethargic. I also had more digestive problems and was gaining weight. After a big meal more blood rushes to stomach for digestion, leaving the brain without the extra oxygenated blood that comes through exercise. This contributed to fatigue. Plus, I was snacking between meals. Now that I've changed my eating habits I have constant energy.

You might try my plan or a modified version of it if you enjoy the pleasure of food as much as I do. It's important to plan your diet and have the proper food available. Do not get in the habit of eating snack or junk foods in this way.

BREAKFAST—EXTENDED OVER 4 HOURS

Food	Amt.	Cal.	Protein(gm)	Fat(gm)	Carbs.(gm)	Sodium(gm)
Grapefruit	1/2	99	12	0.3	22.8	1
Pancakes (4" diam)	3	165	5.4	7.5	19.2	378
Diet maple syrup	3 tbs.	90			23	
Large glass water						
Banana	1	102	1.3	0.3	26.6	1
Oatmeal raisin cookies	4	238	3.2	8	38.6	8.6
Frozen grape juice	8 oz.	135	1	trace	33.0	
Vitamins						
Large glass water						

MIDDAY MEAL—EXTENDED OVER 6 HOURS

Food	Amt.	Cal.	Protein(gm)	Fat(gm)	Carbs.(gm)	Sodium(gm)
Spinach salad	2 c	28	3.6	0.4	4.8	80
Mushrooms for salad	1/2 c	43	2.3	0.7	8	12
Low-cal dressing	1 tbs.	8	trace	0.7	0.4	119
Roast chicken, no skin	3.5 oz.	183	29.5	6.3	0	376
Bread stuffing	1 c	388	8	26	34	1088
Large glass water						
Diet soda						
Baked potato	1 med.	142	4	0.2	32.1	6
Carrots	1 c	45	1.3	0.3	10.4	48
Margarine	2 tbs.	202	0.2	22.6	0.2	276
Water with lime						

EVENING MEAL—EXTENDED OVER 4 HOURS

Food	Amt.	Cal.	Protein(gm)	Fat(gm)	Carbs.(gm)	Sodium(gm)
Split pea soup						
canned, water	1 c	146	8.6	3.2	20.7	272
Crackers-rye wafers	2	45	1.7	0.2	10	116
Large glass water						
Small glass wine	1	137	0.1	trace		trace
Cheese	1 oz.	114	7.1	9.2	0.6	700
Lettuce, tomato,						
onion pieces		36	2	0.2	7.9	11
Wheat bread slices	2	132	4.4	1.2	26.2	266
Water with lemon						
Diet soda						
Apple	1	85	0.5	1	20.5	02
Ice cream	1/2 c	166	1.9	12.0	12	25

Learn the composition of foods so you know which are low in calories, fats and sodium. It can be fascinating.

6) LISTENING TO YOUR BODY

Pain is a sign of trouble. It's our body's way of saying something is wrong. To help avoid problems you should consult your physician before starting on any exercise program. This is especially true if you're over 30, overweight, sedentary, or have any medical problems.

The "no pain/no gain" adage has kept a large number of people from entering an exercise program. Most of us shun pain. Many sports and activities stress certain muscle ligaments and joints so much they cause an abundance of sports-related injuries. My low-stress fitness program is designed to be injury-free.

When to Stop—The following symptoms should prompt you to stop exercising and consult a physician before resuming: abnormal heart action, such as irregular pulse; palpitations in chest or throat, or sudden burst of rapid heartbeats; sudden very slow pulse when a moment before it had been on target; pain or pressure in the center of the chest, arm or throat precipitated by exercise or following exercise.

These disorders may be felt at the time of exercise or after. You should consult a physician who can determine if it constitutes a possible heart problem or a harmless cardiac-rhythm disorder.

If you experience dizziness, lightheadedness, sudden uncoordination, confusion, cold sweat, paleness, blueness or fainting, stop exercising immediately! Lie down with feet elevated until symptoms pass and you can consult a physician.

Body Awareness—Most people who become involved in exercise develop a new body awareness. Our bodies are constantly giving us messages in the forms of anxiety, pain, or feelings of energy and euphoria. As you become more involved in taking good care of yourself, you will be better able to listen to your body. Eventually, your body will indicate when it needs and wants exercise. Exercise produces energy; exercise releases tensions; exercise creates vitality!

You will be able to think of a million excuses each day as to why you shouldn't start your exercises—such as obligations, aches and pains. Our lazy natures will create the excuses. Ignore them and discipline yourself into starting your low-stress activity. If after 15 minutes you feel terrible, worse than when you started, then perhaps you are really fatigued and should stop or slow down.

Plan your exercises so you alternate a vigorous workout one day and an easier workout the next. The hard/easy concept allows for good recovery. Strive for balance.

Aside from checking your pulse, a good way to determine if you are exercising at a comfortable level is the "talk test." If you're able to carry on a conversation with an exercise partner, you are probably not over your target heart rate. If having a conversation becomes difficult, you are close to your target heart rate.

Don't be upset or put off with a few minor aches and pains when you're starting a new exercise program. Deconditioned muscles may be stiff and sore following exercise. During the reconditioning process, the soreness will lessen. Relax those sore muscles in a nice hot bath and be assured that as you become better conditioned you won't be bothered with these discomforts.

7) CONTROLLING MOODS

Exercise has been shown to be effective in relieving mild depression. Some say that adherence to an exercise program gives people a sense of success and makes them feel as if they have accomplished something. This experience makes people feel they have the ability to change. Exercise distracts us from the physical symptoms of depression. We may begin to substitute the positive habits of exercise for their neurotic habits.

This falls in with the "time-out" theory of Dr. William Morgan from the University of Oregon. He suggests that the psychological benefit comes not from the act of exercise itself but from giving the exerciser a chance to get away from stresses. It encourages conscious daydreaming and relaxation. Another theory is that exercise burns up energy that otherwise would produce anxiety.

I have noticed a definite change in my life from exercise. The strength resulting from my training seems to be more mental than physical. That strength means more control over my emotions.

Dr. William Glasser, author of *Positive Addiction,* theorizes that to find happiness, we have to figure out what to do, how to do it and where to get the strength to get it done. Out of the three, he thinks that most people have the most trouble finding strength. Ironically, of the three, it is the easiest to acquire.

Dr. Glasser believes that mentally weak people are most likely to be unhappy because the first response of a weak person is to give up. They tell themselves that they are unable to do whatever is necessary and so quit trying. The second response of the weak is to develop depression, anxiety or psychosomatic illness.

Remember, you create your moods and can control them. Don't allow negative thoughts to enter your mind while working out. Decide to get high on exercise! Once you become conditioned, you'll be able to reach a high because of a tranquilizing chemical let loose in the body during vigorous exercise. I'll discuss that a bit later.

Age and Health—For both men and women, feelings of health and vitality increase with age, even though the incidence of chronic illness also rises. Older people seem to care for themselves better than young people. Older people take more preventive measures, such as setting regular checkups, eating breakfast and getting enough sleep.

Although they participate in fewer sports, people over 60 actually spend more time exercising than those in their 40s and 50s. Older people tend to eat less and better than younger people. Also, older people seem to be more psychologically stable and significantly less neurotic and self-conscious about their bodies than younger people.

Natural Tranquilizer—Morphine-like substances called *endorphins* are released from the pituitary gland. Vigorous exercise can release these hormones, which promote euphoric feelings. Some have called this the reason for "runner's high." Studies show marked increases in the levels of endorphins after very hard exercise, and these feelings can continue for 30 minutes to more than an hour after exercise. High levels of endorphins are present in the body even after moderate exercise, such as those discussed in this book.

Catecholamines are hormones found in the human nervous system. It has been noted that depressed persons have low catecholamine levels. In marathon runners, it was found that catecholamine levels were increased by as much as 300%. During the event these levels returned to normal three or four hours after the race was over.

Mind Control—Studies have shown that a superbly conditioned person is capable of releasing higher levels of endorphins. I can personally attest to the wonder of endorphins and the tremendous power of mind control coping with pain:

I did a stupid thing during the summer of 1984. I decided to ignore a persistent pain in my heel and continued strenuous training. For personal reasons I wanted badly to compete in the U.S. and World Triathlon Championships. And I did.

After the events I went to the doctor. Tests showed that my heel pain was a combination of bone spur, plantar fasciitis and a fractured heel. I had always considered myself a softie who could not tolerate pain. But in the previous six years of exercising and conditioning, I had trained my mind and body to astonishing levels. I have the ability to sometimes turn off pain.

It was during my 12-hour run that I discovered what part our mind plays in coping with pain. About four hours into the event, my knee started to hurt. I checked with some people who were familiar with the type of pain I was experiencing and was assured that I would not do any permanent damage by continuing. Because the majority of my training is done at relaxed, enjoyable levels, I thought it might be good for me to continue even though it wasn't fun anymore. During the next eight hours while I jogged and walked, I refused to let the pain enter my thoughts.

Not once while participating in the four different Ironman Triathlons did I let myself dwell on the fact that I had to cover 140 miles within a 17-hour period. Instead, I would break each event down into small segments my mind could handle without getting depressed. I think that's the way you should look at the low-stress fitness program of this book. Each workout is a small part of the day that you should enjoy.

Mind control is paramount when it comes to endurance events or, for that matter, almost anything in life. The mental aspects of aerobic endurance sports might turn out to be one of psychology's most promising frontiers.

There is an interesting report by two psychologists, Drs. Kobasa and Maddi, from the University of Chicago. They studied the phenomenon of *psychological hardiness*. They wanted to know why some people do not crumble under stress and why they do not become ill under the strain of crisis. They wanted to find out what distinguishing characteristics these people seemed to have. Essentially, the common trait shared by these people were personal attitudes toward challenge, commitment and control. These appear to have a profound effect on health. Stress resides not in the person nor in the situation, but in how people evaluate events.

The researchers also found that a "hardy" personality protects people by decreasing the chances of being ill by as much as 50%. Some people are able to transform events to their advantage and actually seem to thrive in crises.

CHAPTER THREE

Stretching

The relatively new field of *exercise physiology* has given us modern stretching methods based on scientific data. It has been medically proven that stretching is effective in injury prevention and rehabilitation. But for it to be effective, you must stretch properly. Unfortunately, many people seeking fitness are not aware of what is right or wrong.

ESSENTIAL POINTS

1) Never bounce. "Ballistic" stretching can cause microscopic tears in muscle fibers. Scar tissue may then form, causing a gradual *loss* of elasticity.

Also, bouncing can shorten the muscle you are trying to elongate. Your muscles have a protective mechanism called the *stretch reflex*. If you stretch too far or bounce, a nerve reflex tells the muscle to contract to keep it from being injured.

2) Do not stretch to the point of pain. Remember, listen to your body. Pain means something is wrong. Back off if there is pain!

3) Stretching should be easy, relaxing, peaceful and make you feel good. Don't make it a contest or challenge. If stretching is a new experience for you, remember that the aim is *low-stress fitness*. Bodies that were sedentary for years will undoubtedly be less supple in muscles and joints. It will take time to regain youthful flexibility.

HOW TO START

Stretching constitutes an essential part of my personal exercise program. And I'm convinced that it is just as important in your low-stress program. You may prefer to combine it with just one or two, rather than three, of the aerobic activities I suggest. That's fine. Try to make stretching a habit.

Consider stretching a separate activity. I recommend you do it before *and* after participating in any other activity. It will keep you flexible and help prevent injuries. Also, allocate at least one hour a week just for stretching. Are you doubting that you can enjoy an hour of stretching without becoming bored? I'll show you how!

Stretching will improve a body awareness. As you stretch various parts of your body, focus your thoughts on them. It will make you more relaxed and tranquil.

Hold/Relax Method—Some stretching exercises can be done alone, some with a partner or with equipment. Static, easy stretching involves elongating the muscles with no bouncing or forcing. Stretch until you feel a little tightness in the muscle. Then hold the position from 10 to 30 seconds.

As muscle tightness reduces, you then move on to the *developmental* stretch. While still stretched, but relaxed, slowly move a fraction of an inch farther until you feel mild tension. You then hold it for 10 to 30 seconds more.

This combination of moves is called the *hold/relax* method of stretching. It is for relaxing, increasing your range of motion, strength, coordination and flexibility.

Warmup—An important thing to remember is that *before* stretching you must "warm up" muscles and lubricate joints a bit. Your body warms up by pumping blood to muscles and releasing *synovial fluid* to lubricate joints.

Stretching is not the same as warming up. Brisk walking or pedalling a stationary bicycle for 5 to 10 minutes are good ways to increase body temperature and warm up.

Perhaps the quickest and most convenient warmup exercise is the jumping jack. First, stand with your feet together, hands at your sides. Then jump, raising the arms over your head in an arc as you slide both feet shoulder-width apart. Jump back to starting position and repeat. Do 5 or 10 repetitions (reps) per *set* of jumping jacks. Do about three sets, with a short pause between sets until you feel warmed up.

The time to start stretching is when you start to perspire or feel warm. It may take 10 minutes to get adequately warmed up. I remember going to races and watching the way some of the runners did their stretching. They would spend about five minutes of stretching their cold bodies, often using improper movements. Then they would dash off to run the race.

Afterward they would stand around in the cold—or lie on the ground in the summer—and rest for 30 minutes without stretching. No wonder there are so many running injuries!

POST-ACTIVITY STRETCHING

It is very important to stretch again after the main activity. The post-activity stretch, in addition to preventing injury, offers the greatest improvements in flexibility.

After the post-activity stretch, do cool-down. Walk around to allow your body to slowly return to its normal state. This also helps prevent blood from pooling in the legs, which can cause stiffness and soreness.

BREATHING AND POSTURE DURING STRETCHING

I want you to start all of your stretching sessions with a few simple exercises for better breathing and posture. Breathing is the ''art'' of taking fresh air into, and expelling stale air from, the lungs.

Air is one of the important energizers of the human body. (Unfortunately a lot of people are shallow breathers, but this section will help you overcome that problem.) If you are a smoker, you will find my low-stress program to your liking because it is easy and non-stressful. If you consistently follow this exercise program, you will probably want to stop smoking within a year. An exercising body naturally craves proper food, rest and air. People who are exercising have a much easier time giving up smoking than those who do not exercise.

Scientific studies show that the greatest susceptibility to sickness and aging occurs with a breakdown in breathing capability. Other metabolic functions will decline in direct proportion. Without breathing exercises, effective breathing among Americans drops from 100% at birth to roughly 60% during middle age, and to 40% of capacity, or less, during advanced years.

Each time you inhale you are providing blood and nerves with a fresh supply of oxygen. On each exhalation, you are eliminating impurities. Take deep, full breaths when you are exercising. It will take conscious effort at first—you may tend to hold your breath in certain exercises.

BASIC BREATHING

The first two exercises promote proper breathing. Breathe slowly, under control and rhythmically. When doing stretches that call for bending forward, exhale as you bend. Then breathe slowly as you hold the stretch. If your natural breathing pattern is inhibited during a stretch, you are straining too much. Ease up and relax. As mentioned earlier, don't hold your breath when stretching.

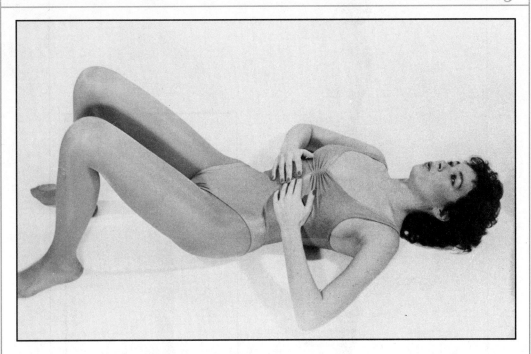

RECLINING BREATHING EXERCISE

As shown above, lie on your back, flat on the floor, with knees bent and feet on floor. Toes should be turned a bit inward. Relax your shoulders and torso. Put your hands, palms down, on your abdomen with tips of middle fingers touching. Keep your elbows on the floor.

Inhale through your mouth to take a deep breath. As your lungs fill with air and the diaphragm descends, allow abdominal muscles to rise.

Exhale slowly. Your rib cage will pull together slightly. Contract abdominal muscles to completely exhale. Repeat five times.

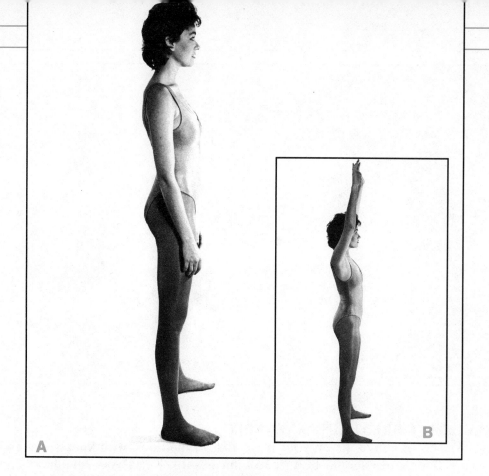

A

B

STANDING BREATHING EXERCISE

As shown in the above series, stand straight, hands at your side, feet shoulder-width apart. Raise your arms straight up, reach over your head and arch backward. Take a deep breath through both nose and mouth and hold it for 5 to 10 seconds.

Then bend forward from the waist as far as possible without bouncing or straining, keeping your knees bent. At the same time, exhale vigorously through the mouth. Let your arms hang between your legs.

The idea is to eventually bring the head below the level of the heart. Compress the chest and push upward with the diaphragm and abdominal muscles to expel all of the air from your lungs.

Now slowly inhale through your nose and mouth. Push downward with your diaphragm and expand your chest at front and sides to draw in the air to the full capacity of your lungs. Inhale as you return to the starting position. Repeat five times.

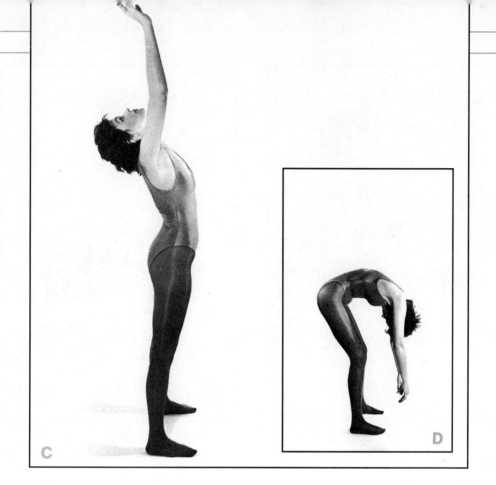

C

D

BASIC POSTURE

Another concern while stretching or exercising is to maintain proper posture. A great number of people have poor posture when sitting, standing and walking. Poor posture can cause backache, neck strain, headache, sciatica, and knee and foot problems. Correcting posture is important because it will definitely make you look and feel better.

There is probably no one best posture for all individuals because body build affects the balance of body parts. But in general, certain relationships are desirable.

Upright Posture—To check your upright posture, stand sideways in front of a full-length mirror or have someone check you from the side. When standing properly, you could hang a plumb line from your earlobe and it would run slightly in front of the shoulder, mid-hip, slightly to the front of the center of the knee and anklebone. Good posture is shown in photo A, page 60.

Your goal is to stand erect and balanced. You should be aligned, symmetrical from side to side and front to back. It will feel strange at first using the ideal position just described, but eventually it will become second nature.

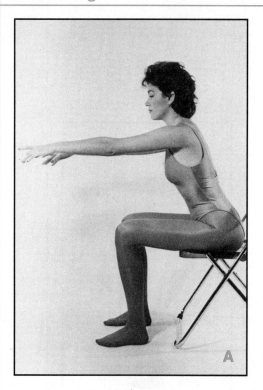
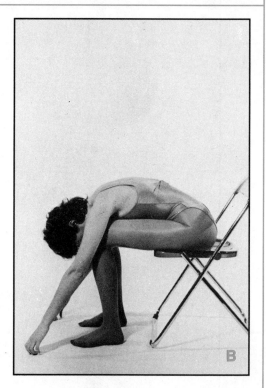

If you allow your head and shoulders to thrust forward, eventually your lower back will hollow out and a belly bulge forms. The result is a dumpy-looking profile. When standing correctly, you'll see that your head "floats" on top of your spine, allowing your chin to ride parallel to the floor.

Keep your shoulders even and relaxed. Let your arms dangle. Slightly lift your breastbone up and out, expanding your chest and narrowing your waist. The pelvis should be lined up under your ribs, with hips even. The legs should swing freely from the hip joints. Your knees should face forward over your feet, toes relaxed.

Practice duplicating this upright posture. No two bodies are alike, so keep in mind that your ideal posture would be the closest position that is reasonably comfortable to that described and pictured here.

PROPER SITTING POSTURE

Desk-bound people should practice correct sitting posture to feel more relaxed at the end of the day. Simply do the following: Avoid slouching. Sit straight rather than lean back. Your bottom should be snug in the back of the chair. Think of your stomach, chest, shoulders, neck and head stacked like building blocks. Feet line up with your knees.

Shown at left is an exercise you can do to improve your sitting posture. Get in the habit of doing it in the middle of your work session:

While seated in a chair, place your feet flat directly below the knees. Reach forward with torso and arms at shoulder level. Press shoulders down, lift abdomen and chest back and up. Next, roll down, reaching out from lower spine. Round your back. Arms and head are hanging.

Breathe deeply five times to loosen up your back muscles. Slowly roll up, inhaling, pressing your abdominals into your spine. Feel the stretch.

At this point, let your arms dangle. Your chest should be lifted, shoulders relaxed, head up and neck loose. Repeat four to eight times.

BASIC STRETCHES FOR MAJOR MUSCLE GROUPS

Now it's time to become better acquainted with various, proper stretches for different muscle groups. I'm going to number the stretches so I can refer to them again later in the chapters on walking, biking and swimming. I'll prescribe a different set of stretches for each activity.

Remember, do some breathing and warmup exercises before stretching. Then go easy on yourself when stretching. You should never go so far as to feel pain.

Don't Forget—Never bounce. Never force yourself by pulling and tugging. When you stretch properly, flexibility will increase. But it takes time. When your body is ready, it will achieve a new range of motion.

Don't compare your flexibility with others, just be concerned with improving your *own* flexibility. You may not be able to achieve the range of motion as described in some stretches, so adapt. For instance, if your toes are out of reach, grasp your ankles or calves instead. You will eventually be able to get to your toes, so be patient, consistent and enjoy yourself.

Useful Advice—The greatest gains in flexibility come with stretching when the muscles are warm. That's why I recommend the pre-stretching warmup described earlier. If you notice that a particular muscle group seems extra tight, spend extra time stretching that area. Concentrate on the muscles you are using. Feel and enjoy the stretch.

It helps to use a rug or mat for your stretching rather than a hard floor. Ideally, stretching exercises should be done once or twice a day. If you can't stretch that often, do it on days of high activity.

When you do standing stretches in which you bend over, as in touching your toes, always have a slight bend in your knees. You will put too much strain on your back with straight legs.

Another bad exercise is the so-called *plow,* the stretch that calls for your feet to be raised up and over your head until your toes touch the floor. This is bad because it compresses vertebrae in the neck. Stay away from that stretch.

Following are the numbered stretching exercises. I assume that you have warmed up, completed your breathing exercises and are ready to start.

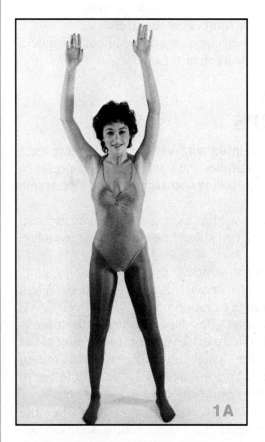
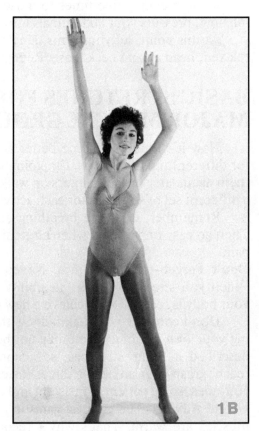

1) STANDING BODY STRETCH

Stand with your feet hip-width apart. Reach with stretched arms toward the ceiling. First lead with the right arm, then with the left. Alternate, doing six on each side.

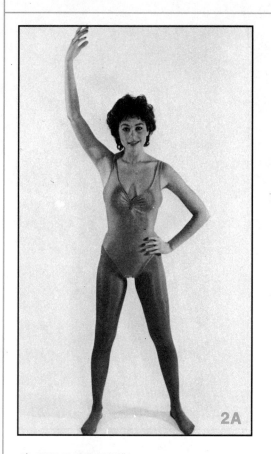

2A

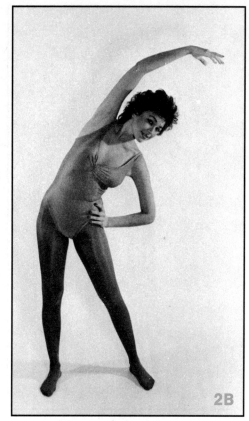

2B

2) SIDE BENDS

Stand with one hand over your head and the other on your hip. Feet should be shoulder-width apart and toes pointed forward. No locked knees—keep them slightly bent. Bend at the waist, slowly to the side with your hand on the hip. Feel the stretch along the side of your arm all the way to your hip. (This is a good stretch for your waistline.) Hold the stretch for about 10 seconds, then relax and do the same on the other side. Do about 15 repetitions.

As shown on the next page, you can increase this stretch by using one arm to pull the other, rather than have it rest on your hip. Gently pull the arm over your head and down toward the ground, being careful not to overstretch.

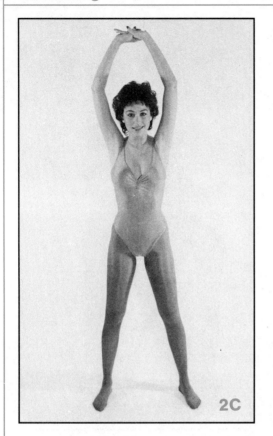

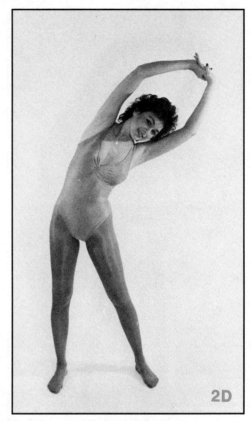

3) HEAD ROLLS

This exercise is shown on the next page. Sit or stand in a comfortable position, keeping your shoulders in an upright, level position. Slowly roll your head from side to side with your chin touching your chest as your head rolls forward. It's not a good idea to roll it backward because of possible damage to the neck over a period of time. If you feel an area that seems extra tight, stop and hold the stretch, but don't strain.

You can do several variations by trying to touch your left ear to the left shoulder. Also try to touch your chin to your shoulder and to your chest. Relax and enjoy the stretching. Do about 15 rotations.

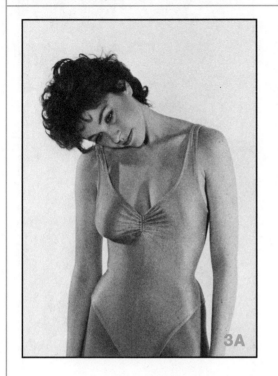

3A

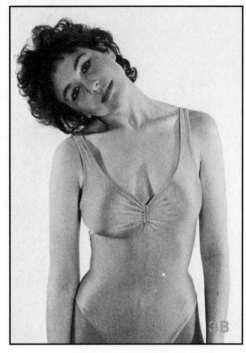

3B

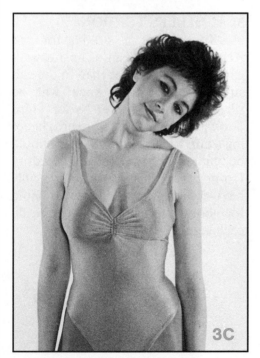

3C

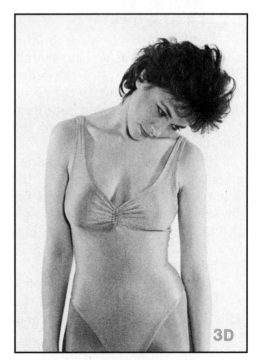

3D

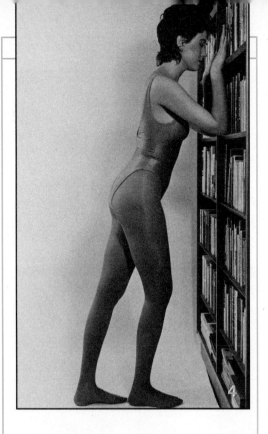

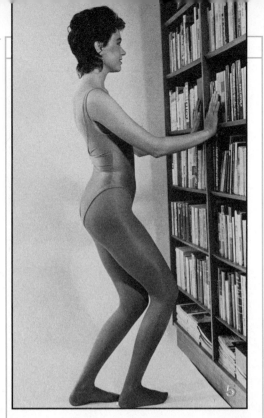

4) CALF MUSCLES

Stand a few feet away from a solid object, such as a chair or wall. Put one foot in front of the other. Bend your arms with forearms on the solid object. Then rest your head on your hands and push with the forearms.

The forward leg is bent and the other leg is straight behind you. It's important to keep the back heel flat on the ground. Keep your lower back flat and slowly move your hips forward. Hold the position for 30 seconds and exhale.

Remember to never bounce when stretching. Do five repetitions with each leg. Feel the stretch in your calf and ankle.

5) ACHILLES TENDON

To achieve a stretch for the Achilles tendon, lean against a wall, with your arms lower than in the calf stretch. Your back knee will be slightly bent. Lower your hips *downward,* rather than forward, keeping your back flat. Your feet should be pointed straight or slightly toed-in. Do not force this as you should only have a slight feeling of stretch. Hold for about 20 seconds. Be sure to do each leg.

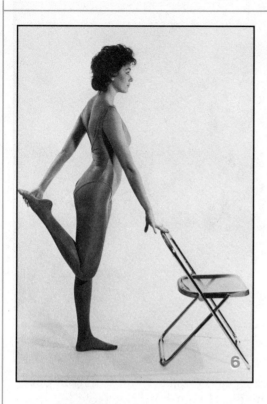

6) STORK STRETCH FOR QUADRICEPS AND KNEES

While you have the wall or chair for support, stretch your *quads* and knees. *Quadriceps* are the large, front thigh muscles, located between knee and hip. These muscles stabilize the knee and are used in lifting the leg. They are composed of four parts, all of which are generally known as the "quads."

For this stretch you are standing on one leg supporting yourself by leaning against a tree or wall. Lift your leg behind you, bending it at the knee. Hold onto your foot with the hand from the opposite side, right foot/left hand or left hand/right foot. You will see a lot of people doing this stretch with the same-side hand holding the foot. I recommend the opposite because that lets your knee bend at a natural angle.

Never stretch the knee to the point of pain. You must be careful in stretching quads, especially if you have had knee problems. Hold the stretch for about 20 seconds and repeat with the other leg. Do four or five repetitions.

You may find this too difficult at first. Don't worry, I'll give you an easier quad stretch. But before long you'll be able to do this one and look like a stork!

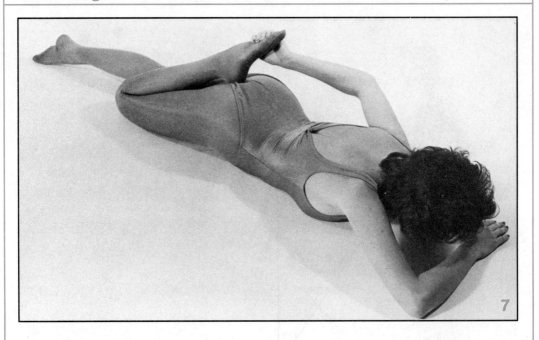

7) STOMACH/LEG STRETCH

Lie face down on the floor. Bend one leg and grasp the foot with your opposite hand. Gently pull the foot toward middle of your buttocks. Hold for about 10 seconds. Do five repetitions. Switch to the other leg. Do five repetitions.

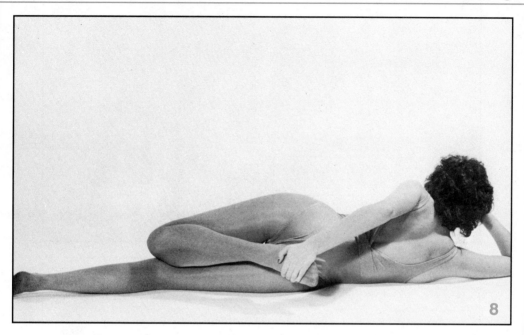

8

8) SIDE QUAD AND LEG STRETCH

Lie on your right side and rest your head on your right hand. Grasp your left foot with your left hand. Gently attempt to touch the heel to the buttock. Hold a relaxed stretch for 10 seconds. Do five repetitions on each side.

I'll soon explain a few ways to stretch quads while sitting on the floor. For now, I want you to concentrate on the quads to be sure you're stretching the correct muscle. Be particularly aware of any knee pain in this exercise. If you have a problem, stretch your quads by doing the stork stretch, #6.

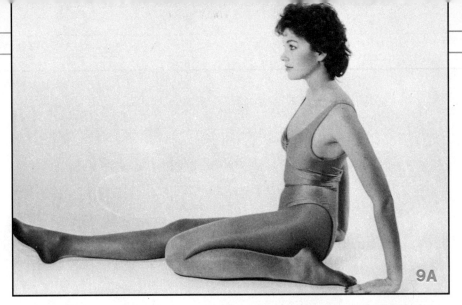

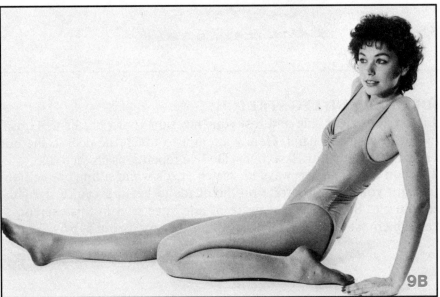

9) SITTING QUAD STRETCH

Sit down and bend your left knee, placing your left heel to the outside of your left hip. Your right leg can be either straight out in front of you or bent with the sole of the right foot next to the inside of your upper left leg. The left foot should be pointed straight back. If it points to the side, you will be putting stress on the knee. Your arms are at your sides for balance. Slowly lean straight back until you feel an easy stretch. Don't let your left knee raise off the floor. Hold the stretch for about 20 seconds.

DEVELOPMENTAL STRETCHES

When you are acquainted and comfortable with the stretches just described and feel complete control, you can start doing the *developmental stretch*. That's where you move a fraction of an inch farther until you feel a mild tension. Hold the tension between 10 and 30 seconds, according to your conditioning. Breathe fully and stay in control. If the tension does not diminish some, ease off slightly. Be sure to switch sides with all stretches.

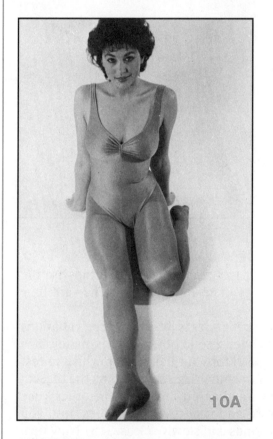

10A

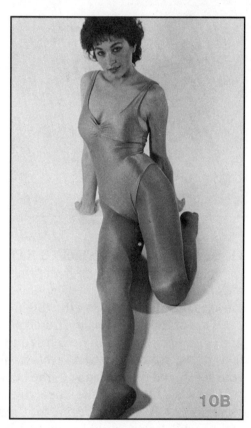

10B

10) FRONT OF HIP AND UPPER THIGH

While in this same position as #9, try tensing the buttocks on the side of the bent leg as you turn the hip toward the opposite leg. This will give a better overall stretch to the upper thigh area and front of the hip. Contract the buttocks for five to eight seconds and then relax. Drop your hip down and continue to stretch the quad for another 15 seconds.

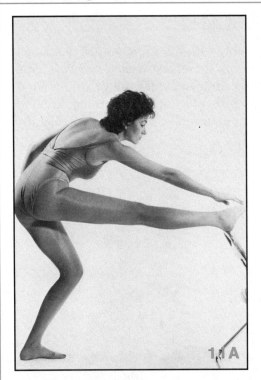
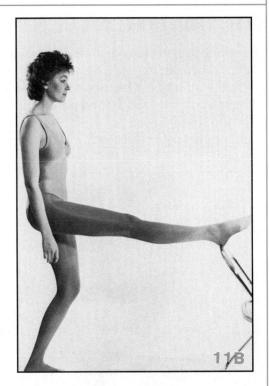

11) STANDING HAMSTRING STRETCH

It's best to stretch the hamstrings after the quadriceps. Hamstrings are the muscles at the back of your leg between the knee and buttocks. They are four muscles that flex the leg on the thigh.

One of the best ways to stretch all these muscles is by doing three variations of the *standing hamstring* stretch. You will need a solid object approximately two feet off the ground—or at a comfortable level for your height—on which to rest your leg. Stand on one leg with the heel of the other leg supported by the object.

Now slightly bend the knee you are standing on, but keep the other knee straight. (A) Turn the bottom foot inward and lean toward the toes until you feel a good stretch. Hold for about 12 seconds and slowly release. (B) Now turn your toes straight up and lean forward again. Hold for 12 seconds then relax. (C) Then turn your foot outward and repeat the movement.

You should be able to feel the stretch in separate muscles of your hamstring with the different toe positions. Do about five repetitions with each leg.

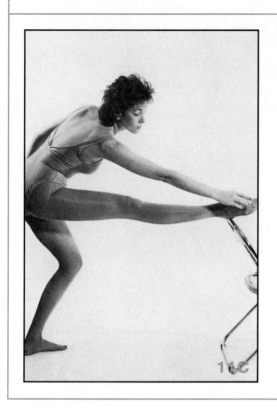

11C

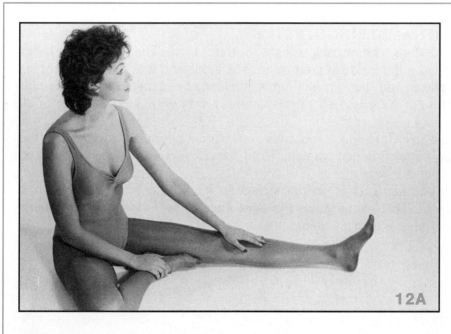

12A

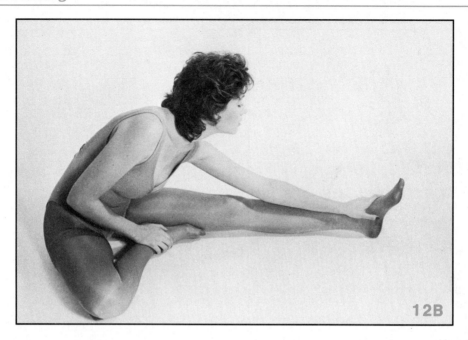

12B

12) SITTING HAMSTRING STRETCH

Sit on the floor with one leg straight in front of you. The sole of your other foot should touch the inside of your thigh. The ankle and toes of the straight leg should be relaxed and the foot held upright. Slowly bend forward from the hips toward the foot of the straight leg until you feel a very slight stretch. Hold for 20 seconds.

After the stretch feeling has diminished, bend a bit more forward from the hips for the developmental stretch. Hold for 25 seconds. Switch sides and stretch the opposite side.

Be sure you don't try to do this stretch in the hurdler's position with one leg behind you. That would place the bent knee in an awkward position and could cause strains or torn ligaments.

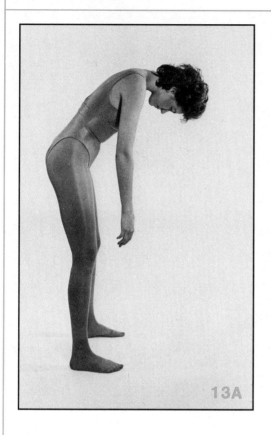
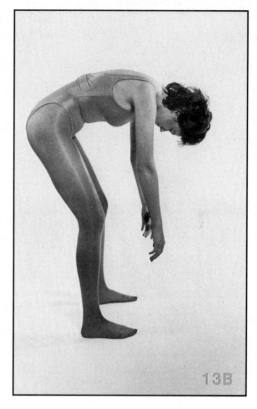

13A

13B

13) FORWARD BEND

This stretch is for the hamstrings, lower back, hips and groin. It is important to keep knees slightly bent. If you do this exercise with straight legs, you are taking the chance of straining your hamstrings and back by trying to stretch already-contracted muscles.

Stand with feet about shoulder-width apart and pointed straight ahead. Slowly bend forward from the hips. Keep your neck and arms relaxed, and let them hang. Do not try to touch the floor or your toes right away. When you feel the first slight stretch in the back of your legs, stay in this easy phase for 15 to 25 seconds and relax. You will gradually loosen up and be able to touch the floor. Never bounce.

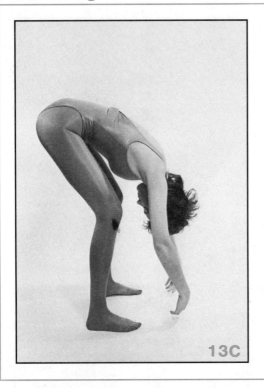

13C

14) GROIN STRETCH

Sit on the floor and put the soles of your feet together with your heels a comfortable distance from your crotch. Your hands should be holding your toes and feet. Try to keep your elbows on the outside of your lower legs during the stretch. You are going to gently pull forward until you feel a good stretch in your groin, the area inside your upper thighs.

Don't start the movement from your head and shoulders. That will put pressure on your lower back. Keep your lower back flat and bend from the hips. Look forward, concentrate on bending from the hips rather than shoulders.

Now carefully move your upper body forward until you feel an easy stretch in the groin area. Remember to start with an easy stretch for 20 seconds, then very slightly increase the stretch into a developmental stretch for 20 seconds. Be careful not to overstretch. Do not make any jerky, bouncing or quick movements.

Do a variation of this stretch by sitting against a wall for support. Keep your back straight and the soles of your feet together. With your hands on the inside of your thighs above the knees, not on them, gently push down until you get a good even stretch. Hold for 20 seconds and relax.

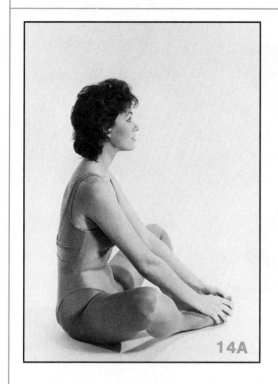

14A

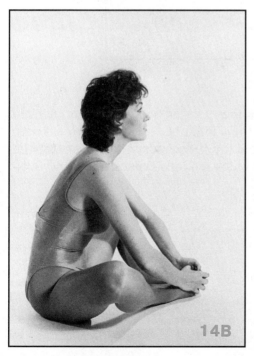

14B

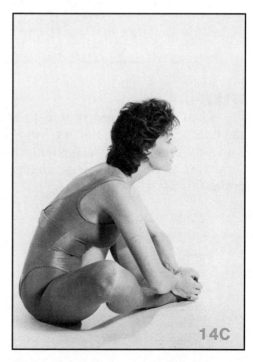

14C

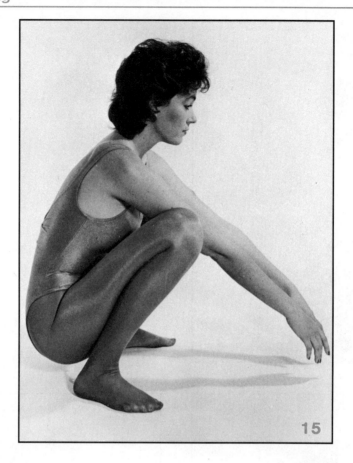

15

15) SQUAT

Squat down keeping your feet flat and toes pointed out. Keep your knees to the outside of your shoulders. Your big toe should be right under your knees with arms dangling between your legs. Hold for 30 seconds. This will stretch the front part of your lower legs, ankles, Achilles tendons, knees, back and deep groin.

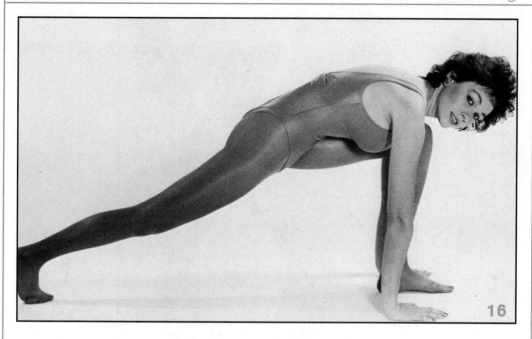

16

16) ILIOPSOAS LUNGE

Crouch down on one leg with the other leg extended behind you. The knee of the forward leg should be directly over your ankle. The other knee can be resting on the floor or on the toes of the back foot. Use your hands for support by placing them on the floor outside your legs. Slowly lower the front of hip downward to create an easy stretch. Hold for 30 seconds. Do both sides.

This is a stretch for the front of your hip, or *iliopsoas*. You may also feel it in the groin and hamstrings. It's good for lower-back problems. If you feel pain in your knee, refrain from the stretch.

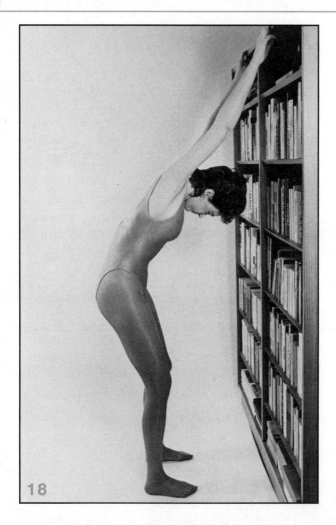

18

17) STANDING UPPER-BODY AND BACK STRETCH

You will need to hang on to something for this exercise. A cabinet, the re-frigerator or a ledge will work. Stand away from the ledge with your hands shoulder-width apart and resting on it. Let your upper body drop down. Be sure your hips are directly above your feet and knees slightly apart. Hold the stretch for about 25 seconds. This is a good stretch for a tired upper back that has been slumping over a desk all day.

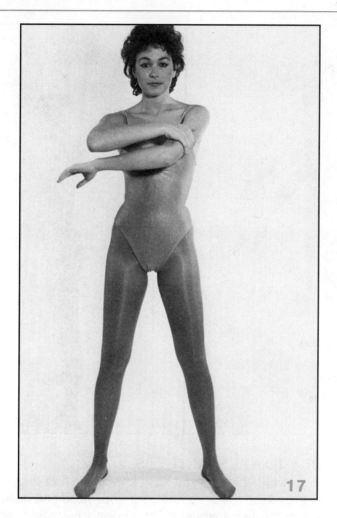

17

18) HOLD/RELAX STRETCH FOR UPPER BODY

Stand up straight. With your right hand, hold the left arm above the elbow on the outside. Move the arm to the left until you feel a tightness. Use the muscles in the upper back and slowly increase the strength of those contractions. Attempt to hold up the left arm away from the right hand, which is offering immovable resistance. Inhale, hold for five seconds, then exhale and relax. Move the left arm farther toward the right side to a new point of tightness, and repeat the exercise. Do five repetitions and switch to the other arm.

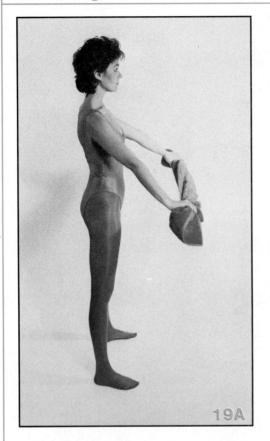
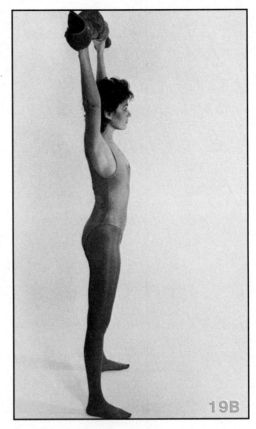

19A

19B

19) UPPER-BODY TOWEL STRETCHES

Hold a rolled towel, which should be at least three feet long, near the ends. You are going to move the towel up and over your head and down behind your back while keeping your arms straight. If you don't have free movement, you may need a longer towel and have to move your hands farther apart because you don't want to strain or force the stretch. Go slowly and feel the stretch.

You can isolate the feeling in certain tight and sore areas by holding the stretch. When you become more flexible, you will be able to hold the towel with your hands closer together. Get in the habit of taking a few minutes when you get out of the shower to do these stretches.

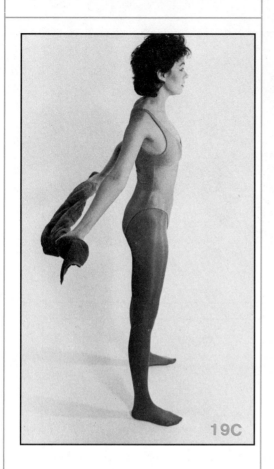

19C

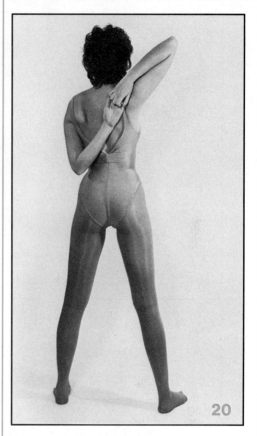

20

20) SHOULDER STRETCH

Reach behind yourself with the right arm over the top of the right shoulder. Your left arm is behind you, palm out. Try to grasp one hand with the other. You may find that your hands can't reach each other, or they can in just one direction. If that's a problem, drop a towel behind your head. With the upper arm bent, reach up with the other arm and grab the towel. Slowly move your hand up on the towel, pulling your upper arm down. As you become more limber, your hands will eventually meet.

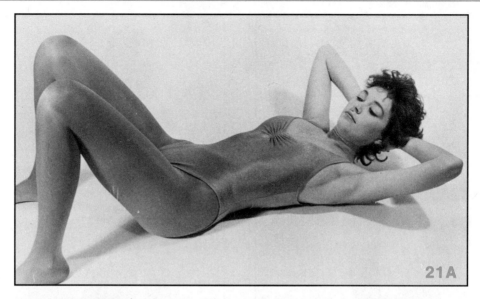

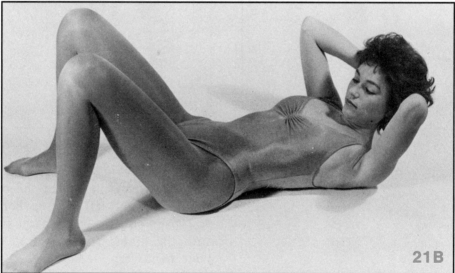

21) UPPER SPINE AND NECK

This stretch will reduce tension in the neck area and loosen up the upper spine and neck. Lie on the floor with your knees bent. Connect your fingers behind your head at ear level. Using the power of your arms, slowly pull your head forward until you feel a slight stretch in the back of your neck. Hold for 5 to 10 seconds and slowly lower your head to the floor. Do three to five repetitions.

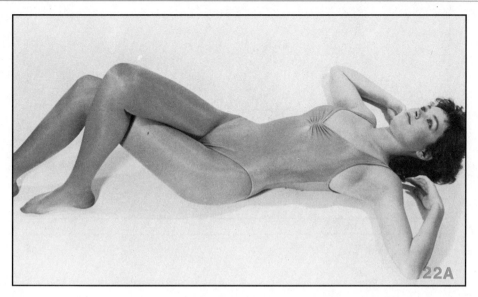

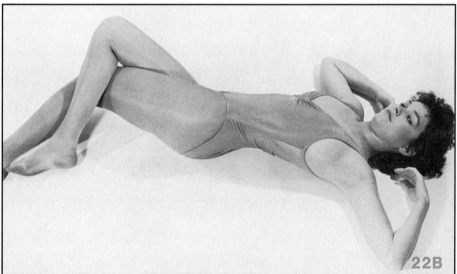

22) LOWER BACK, TOP OF HIP AND SIDE

This is a good stretch if you have *sciatic* problems—problems with a nerve in the upper leg. Assume the same position as in the previous exercise, except keep your head and arms on the floor. Lift the right leg over the left leg. Now use the right leg to pull the left leg toward the floor. Keep the back of your head, upper back, shoulders and elbows flat on the floor.

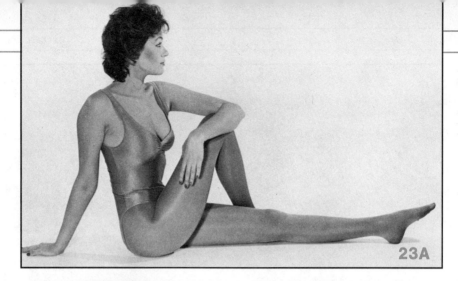

23A

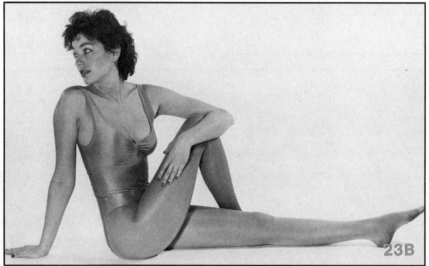

23B

23) SPINAL TWIST

Sit with your left leg straight, bend your right leg and place that foot to the outside of your left knee. Bend your left elbow and rest it to the outside of your upper right thigh, just above the knee.

Use the elbow to keep the leg stationary with controlled pressure to the inside. Your right hand should be resting behind you. Slowly rotate your upper body toward your right arm and look over your right shoulder. Hold for 15 seconds. Do several repetitions on each side.

This stretch is good for your lower back and hips. It is also beneficial for your rib cage and upper back.

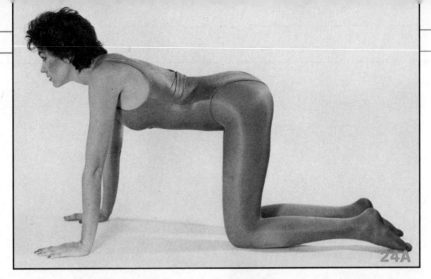

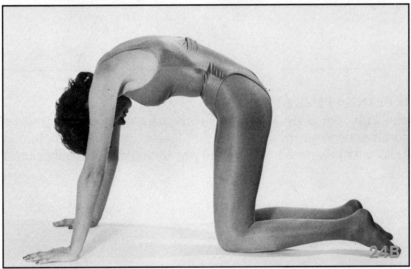

24) CAT BACK

This stretch is for the lower back. Kneel on all fours with arms slightly farther apart than shoulder width. Legs are close together. Start with your back straight and then arch it as high as possible, raising your back towards the ceiling. Pause after each repetition and exhale. Do five times.

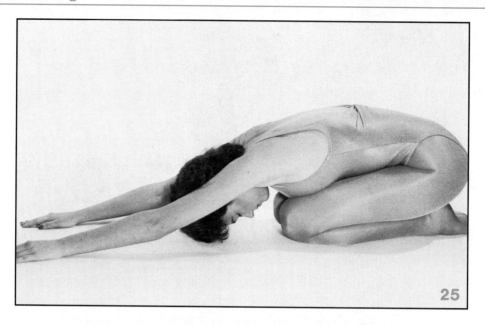

25

25) KNEELING SPINE STRETCH

Kneel with your chest lowered to your thighs. Legs are tucked under you and arms stretched out in front. Breathe deeply. Feel the stretch in arms and spine. Relax with this stretch. It's a good way to unwind and reduce tension.

26) PELVIC TILT

Lie on your back with knees bent, feet flat on the floor. Pinch buttocks together to press small of back against floor. Roll pelvis up toward ceiling. Hold for 5 to 10 seconds and relax. Repeat seven times. This stretch can aid in correcting sway back, and stretches the muscles in the lower back.

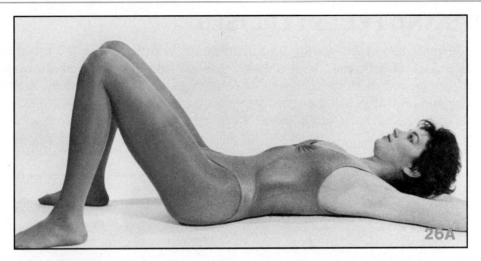

26A

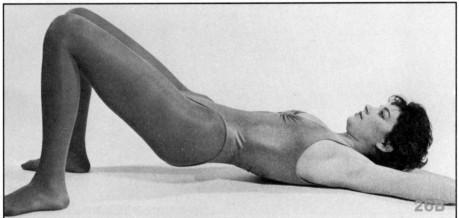

26B

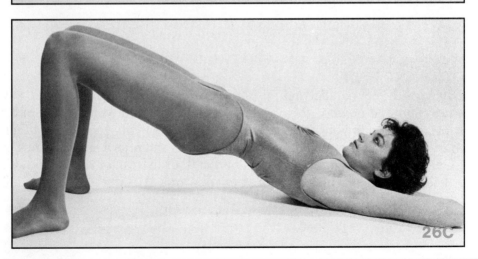

26C

LEG AND FEET EXERCISES

When I taught ice skating I was constantly hearing people tell me about weak ankles. Usually the "weak ankles" resulted from poorly fitted skates that gave no support. I devised a series of exercises to strengthen feet, arches, ankles and legs. If you're not used to walking a lot or being on your feet, you would be wise to learn to do them. Work up to about 12 repetitions of each exercise.

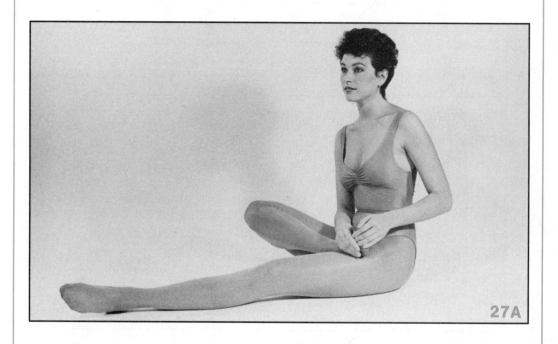

27A

27) TOES AND FEET

Stand with feet parallel and raise toes upward as far as possible and slowly return to floor. Sit down with your legs crossed in front of you. Gently pull the toes toward you with your fingers to stretch the top of your foot and tendons of the toes. Hold an easy stretch for about 10 seconds and repeat several times.

Get some marbles and place them on the floor in front of you. While sitting in a chair, pick the marbles up with your toes, one at a time. Twist your ankle and deposit them in another pile.

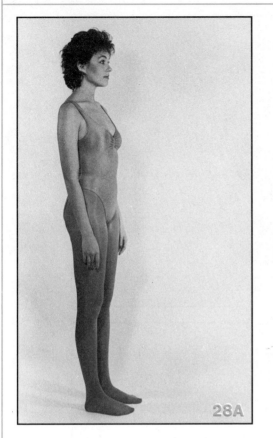

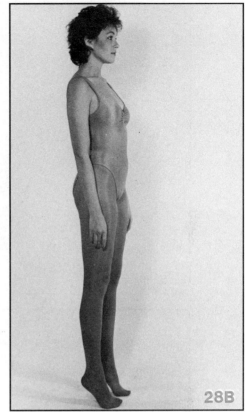

28) ARCHES

Stand with your feet pointing straight ahead about six to eight inches apart. Rise on your toes and then slowly, to the count of 10, return to starting position.

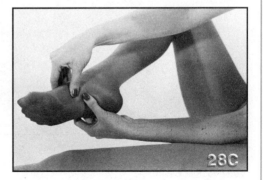

While sitting, massage the longitudinal arch of your foot up and down with your thumbs. Apply a good amount of pressure, using circular motions. This will loosen the tissues and relax your feet.

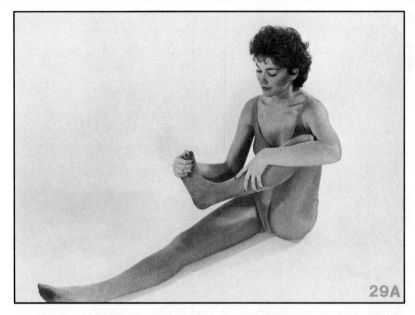

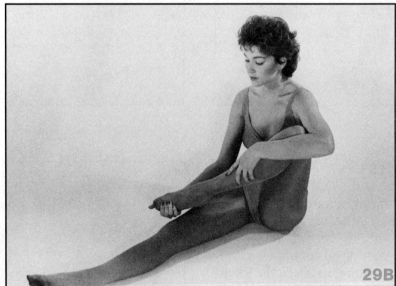

29) ANKLES

Sitting with one leg crossed in front of you, rotate the ankle of the crossed leg clockwise and counterclockwise through a complete range of motion. You should provide a slight resistance with your hand. This is a good exercise to stretch tight ligaments. Stretch both ankles.

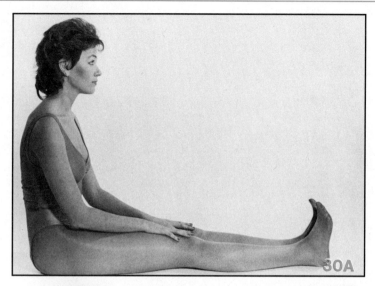

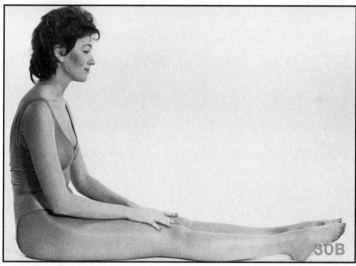

30) CALF AND HEEL

Sit with both legs straight ahead. Bend your feet upward as far as you can, then point them straight forward. In the same position, make circles with your feet in a clockwise and counterclockwise position.

Try and get in the habit of doing stretching and strengthening exercises in conjunction with something you normally do, such as brushing your teeth, washing or sitting at your desk. For example, these are good exercises to do while watching TV.

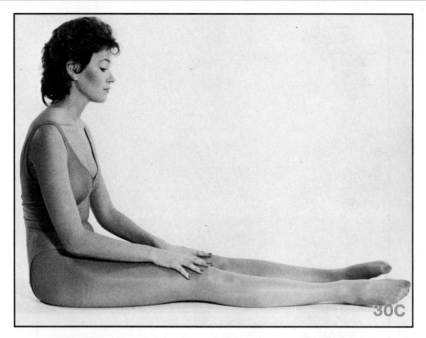

30C

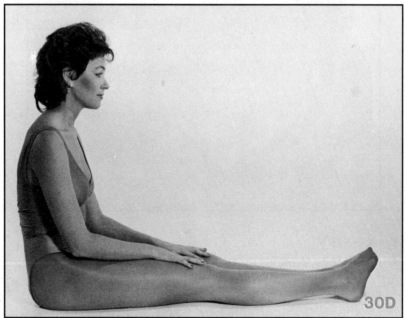

30D

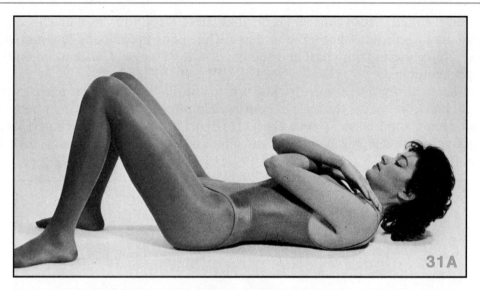

31A

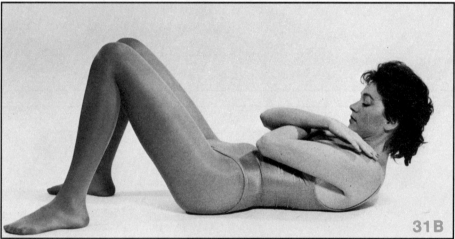

31B

31) ABDOMINALS

Sit-ups are usually considered the best exercise for strengthening abdominal muscles. Often they are done quickly in a jerking motion, with too many repetitions. Done that way they can cause back or neck strain. Also, straight-leg sit-ups can be bad for your lower back. Your abdominal muscles can raise your body off the floor to about a 30° angle. If you raise farther, you will activate the primary hip flexor muscles attached to the lower back. This puts severe stress there.

To avoid back injury, do abdominal curls with your shoulder blades off the floor at no more than a 30° angle. Lie on your back with your knees bent, feet flat on the floor. Cross your hands on your chest. Keep your head in a fixed position and don't let it bob up and down. Curl your upper body forward with your chin close to your chest and shoulders at a 30° angle. Concentrate on the upper abdominals.

Then slowly lower your back down to the floor. When you uncurl your upper and lower body, the back of your head should not touch the floor because your chin should be near your chest. Do 5 or 10 of these at medium speed, working on developing body rhythm. Think about the muscles being used in this exercise.

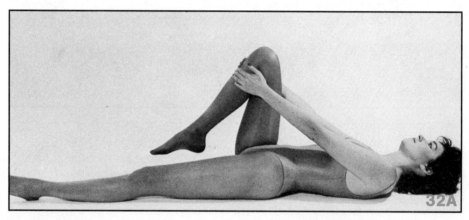

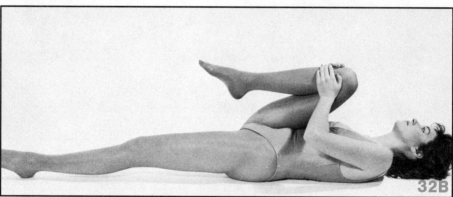

32) WILLIAMS I & II

Lie flat on your back on the floor. One leg is outstretched, the other knee is raised to your chest. Your hands are hugging your bent leg on the upper part of the shin. Move the leg as close to your shoulder as comfortable. Do five repetitions with each leg.

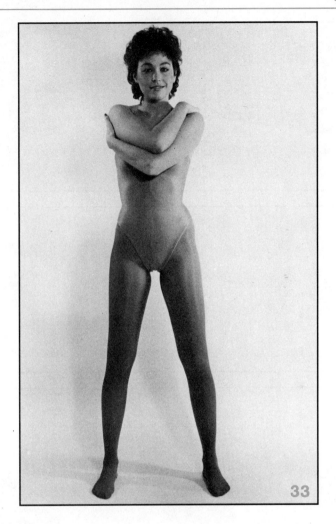

33) UPPER BACK HUG

You're doing so well with your stretching that I'd like to give you a hug. But since I can't, give yourself one. Actually that's just the way to do this exercise for your upper back. While standing up straight, cross your arms across your chest. With one hand on top of your shoulder and the other under your arm, reach as far back on you back as possible. Inhale as you squeeze tightly with both hands. Exhale and say, "I love me." Do five repetitions, then switch position of hands and repeat.

My son was doing this exercise with his girlfriend watching. Finally, she said, "I love you too," and started hugging him. This could become your favorite stretch. It's good for the ego too.

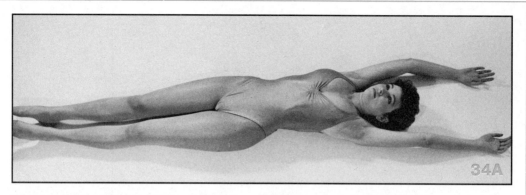

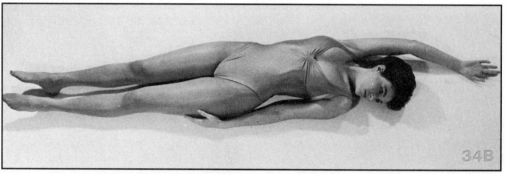

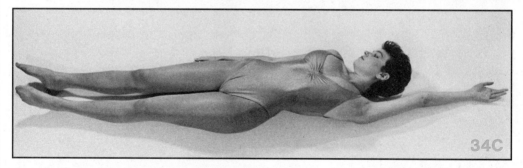

34) OVERALL BODY STRETCH

Lie flat on the floor with your legs together and toes pointed and stretch your arms overhead at shoulder width. This is a two-way stretch, so reach in opposite direction with your arms and legs. Hold the stretch for five seconds, relax and exhale. Another variation of this is a diagonal stretch. In the same position, reach with the toes of your right foot as you reach with your left arm.

Hold for five seconds and then relax. Proceed with the opposite side. This is a very relaxing stretch. You'll feel the effect in various muscle groups. Do this stretch to reduce tension and tightness. It will relax your spine and entire body.

CHAPTER FOUR

Walking

You may wonder why a marathoner and Ironwoman has written a book advocating walking rather than jogging or running. The answer is simple—I have learned that I can get the same benefits from brisk walking as from running. And without bodily stress!

This is important, as shown by a recent survey taken by *Runner's World* magazine. It reported that 6 out of 10 runners were disabled at least part of the year by injuries.

Other research has shown that whether you run, jog, run and walk—or just walk three miles—you gain the same fitness benefits, if your pace is at least 15 minutes per mile.

RUNNING VS. WALKING

Running injuries can be attributed to the fact that few people possess a runner's body. Running experts say that a good long-distance runner should weigh only two pounds for every inch of height. *Ectomorphs,* a body type characterized by thin bones and muscles, have the runner's body and are less prone to injury.

Dr. George Sheehan writes, "Only 10% to 15% of people are natural runners . . . Running is suitable exercise for a rather small group of people; walking, however, is recommended for nearly everyone . . . The runner and walker are entirely different. The runner is concerned with the conquering of space and time. He runs with a goal and purpose, preparing himself for the ultimate effort, trying to reach his own perfection.

"All of this calls for constant attention, to breathing, arm movement, rhythm . . . Only through this unnatural awareness can he attain the classical yet instinctual form of the champion.

"The walker is past all this. For him, observation and thoughts dominate. His qualifications, according to Emerson, include vast curiosity, good speed, good silence and an eye for nature. The walker looks for enough to feed the human spirit for a single day."

Dr. Sheehan continues, "If this suggests that walkers are mature men *(sic)* with a capacity for observation, men with empathy for their environment, it is because it always has been so. Where all other athletes must be in attention to the way they move, the walker can retire into a reverie of complete detachment. The walker has found the peace that the runner still seeks."

Walking Physiology—Running and jogging jolt and jar joints, bones and muscles. As we jump from one foot to the other in running, all our weight lands on one foot.

Walking is not a jumping motion. Rather, it is a smooth progression of steps. The rear foot does not leave the ground until the advancing foot has touched down. There is no jolt because there is no quick transfer of weight from one foot to another.

The runner is literally falling onto each foot from a higher point above the ground than is the walker, so the runner's foot is hitting the ground with much more force.

The beauty of walking is that it's one of the easiest, most natural, graceful and mildest of exercises. No one set of muscles runs the risk of being overtaxed. It's almost impossible to walk too much.

WALKING IS FOR EVERYBODY

Charles T. Kinzleman, who has a doctorate in exercise physiology, is national fitness consultant to the YMCA and author of many books on health and fitness. He states, "Running is not for everyone. For some people it is too strenuous, too demanding. For some it's a hassle. Many people take up running and soon stop. For all these ex-joggers and ex-runners, I submit that walking is the perfect exercise."

Walking is for everyone—the young and old, male and female, sick and healthy. You can walk to work, the store, in parks, the woods, to explore cities, along beaches and streams. You can walk alone, with friends, a dog or a lover. You can feel the wind, the personality of a neighborhood, new seasons, the texture of air, feel the different inflections of sand, soil, rock and asphalt.

Considering all of this, it's no wonder that walking is the American's main source of exercise. The human body is perfect for walking. We are better constructed for walking than for sitting, standing or running because of the

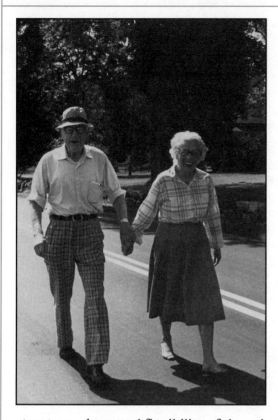

Walking is good for every body. This chapter shows how it's one of the foundations of a low-stress exercise plan.

structure, shape and flexibility of the spine. It is the ideal low-stress activity.

The Second Heart—The leg muscles are often referred to by cardiologists as the "second heart." The circulatory system of human beings has to deal with the force of gravity. Unlike four-legged animals that have all vital organs on about the same level, humans need to move their blood back to their hearts despite the pull of gravity. The muscles below the waist, in our abdomen, buttocks, thighs, calves and feet compose this "second heart." They help pump blood back to the heart.

One of the reasons doctors prescribe walking for recuperating heart patients is because it's one of the best ways to make the lower muscles do their share of the work. Prolonged sitting or standing causes blood to pool in the lower extremities. This slows the return rate and volume of blood and forces the heart to work harder. Walking contracts calf, thigh and buttocks muscles, which helps to squeeze blood back up toward the heart. The heart must work harder when it doesn't receive this help from the legs.

Walking can lower blood pressure and heart rate by improving circulation. It can also be beneficial in preventing phlebitis and varicose veins. We have to keep blood moving, especially when you consider that within a 24-hour period our circulatory system pushes 1,900 gallons of blood through nearly hundreds of miles of circulatory byways!

G. M. Trevelyan says, "I have two good doctors—my right leg and my left." If we use them consistently in brisk walking we can improve our health. Dr. Paul Dudley White, the late, eminent cardiologist, said, "A minimum of an hour a day of fast walking is absolutely necessary for one's optimal health, including that of the brain." He also said, "Walking is as natural as breathing."

Walking briskly increases your oxygen transport capacity, the amount of oxygen that each heartbeat delivers to the rest of the body. We improve mental alertness when larger amounts of oxygen are delivered to the brain cells through exercise.

The Perfect Exercise—Health and medical authorities recommend walking as an excellent exercise, with a wealth of benefits. Our muscles and tissues are strengthened through exercise as they stretch, turn and knead with every step we take. A large majority of our muscles are used when we walk, especially if we swing our arms. Complexions can improve from the fresh air and increased blood flow. Walking can aid digestion, elimination and sleep. Studies have shown walking to be beneficial to sufferers of migraine headaches, menstrual discomfort and emphysema.

Walking, the mildest, easiest sport, is the best way for the obese, the senior citizen or the cardiac patient to get back in shape.

If You Have Arthritis or Heart Problems—The American Arthritis Foundation also considers walking a good exercise. It is estimated that at least 50 million Americans have some form of arthritis. These people can often benefit from a program of walking, but should proceed cautiously, as should those who are obese or are victims of heart disease.

A balance is needed between rest and exercise, which will vary depending on the severity of the arthritis or heart problem. With arthritis, joints should be moved gently each day. An arthritic person who hasn't been exercising regularly may be surprised and pleased to see the progress he can make in a few months of regular, low-stress walking.

If You Have Blood-Sugar Problems—Dr. Fred W. Whitehouse, president of the American Diabetes Association said, "As exercise lowers the blood sugar, it follows that exercise should help control diabetes, which it does."

He advises, "Never hesitate to exercise; just adjust to it. Benefits of exercise go far beyond helping to control diabetes. Exercise has a true effect on the body. Your muscle tone improves; your sense of well-being and self-esteem grow. Your weight is easier to control; your step is lighter; your breath comes easier; general tension decreases."

Psychological Benefits—There are also great psychological benefits to be derived from walking. A combination of pleasant thoughts and exercise helps get

STRETCHES FOR WALKING

Exercise #	Name
1	Standing Body Stretch
2	Side Bends
4	Calf Muscle
5	Achilles Tendon
6	Stork Stretch
7	Stomach/Leg Stretch
11	Standing Hamstring Stretch
12	Sitting Hamstring Stretch
13	Forward Bend
14	Groin Stretch
16	Iliopsoas Lunge
27	Toes and Feet
28	Arches
29	Ankles
30	Calf and Heel

rid of anxiety. Dr. Herbert A. deVries of the Gerontology Center of the University of Southern California finds that a vigorous 15-minute walk reduces neuromuscular tension more effectively than 400mg of a common tranquilizer.

Regular vigorous walking is nature's antidote for stress and strain. We can escape—not only from the madness of the world but from our own immediate pressures. Occasionally we need to escape from those near and dear to us too—our partners, children or parents.

Even if we can't walk away from our problems or worries, we can often walk them off and return feeling bolstered and rejuvenated. Walking has been shown to improve morale, productivity, creativity and intellect. Walking can provide an outlet for pent-up emotions, while ideas fall into place.

Psychologist Gene Boyko recommends walking to relieve stress. He walks often because his teaching position confines him to rectangular rooms with a lot of hard, straight lines. He takes his walks in the woods where there are no straight lines!

Literary and Historical Attitudes—Through the ages people were relieved of stress or escaped from it through walking. This poem by Edna St. Vincent

Millay tells of that carefree feeling:

Departure

It's little I care what path I take
And where it leads it's little I care. . .
I wish I could walk for a day and a night
and find me a dream in a desolute place
With never the rut of a road in sight
Nor the roof of a house, nor the eyes of a face.

Robert Louis Stevenson said, "I travel not to go anywhere, but to go."

Fifth-century B.C. Greeks believed that walking made their mind lucid and helped them crack problems of logic and philosophy. Hippocrates believed that long walks were a good tonic for healthly living.

Other poets and philosophers have advocated walking. Emerson said, "Tis the best of humanity that comes out to walk."

Henry David Thoreau wrote of Walden, "But no weather interfered with my walks, or rather my going abroad, for I frequently trampled eight or ten miles through the deepest snow."

Aristotle, Sigmund Freud and Albert Einstein were avid walkers too.

One Woman's Experience—Betty Dolen of Ridgefield, Connecticut, "famous" within her family, is a person you should know about. She likes to walk. And in the early years of her marriage, when she just had three children, she would bundle them into the buggy for her daily treks.

As more children arrived, her daily walks became impossible, until one day about 18 years ago when she read Dr. Kenneth Cooper's first book on aerobics. She became intrigued with walking a measured mile. So she measured off her back yard and walked back and forth to complete a mile. On rainy days she would walk a measured mile in her basement.

Then a friend mentioned that eight times around the local baseball field was a mile, so she put her children in the middle of the field while she walked. You'll hear more about Betty Dolen, nicknamed the *Happy Hoofer,* at the end of the book when I tell you about where these exercises can lead.

EQUIPMENT BEFORE YOU START

I want to get you walking so you can experience the benefits you have been reading about. The first great aspect of walking is that it requires very little equipment. However, a good pair of shoes is very important. Our feet consist of 26 bones intricately linked by 33 joints and tied together with 200 ligaments. They deserve respect an comfort.

The Right Walking Shoe—Here's an adage you must remember before buying shoes: *Cheap shoes may save you money; but high-quality shoes will save your feet.*

I strongly recommend buying your shoes at a store specializing in running shoes. Ideally, the salesperson will inquire about your needs and then offer a wide selection. Try on several different brands and walk around the shop to try out the various pairs. Your feet are unique. Only you can determine which pair feels best.

Keep the following in mind when selecting your shoes:

● There should be at least a quarter or half inch of room ahead of your big toe in the front of the shoe.

● You should be able to wiggle and spread out your toes without rubbing.

● When you walk, your foot will slide forward inside the shoe. Any pressure on the front or side of the shoe can cause blisters or cramped toes.

● The shoes you select should have a lot of cushioning on the heels and soles. Running shoes will provide that cushioning to absorb the shock. Do not buy a racing shoe. Instead, ask for a training shoe. It offers more cushion.

● Most good shoes have double soles—a tough outer layer to resist impact and provide traction, and one or more softer layers inside to cushion feet and absorb shocks.

Generally, a good running shoe is also a good walking shoe. Even so, there are many different brands, designs and styles to choose among. Spend the necessary time and money to get a shoe that's comfortable and usable on all types of terrain. Photo courtesy of Saucony.

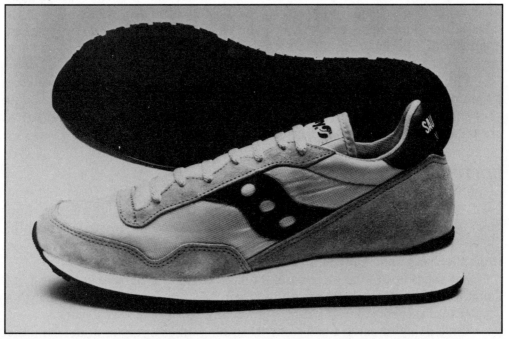

• The heel should be moderately elevated, and the shoe should hold the heel of the foot snug, without discomfort. Check the shoe to be sure the top of the heel touches the back of your foot at a comfortable level. If it's too high, you may develop tendon problems or blisters. If it is too low, there will not be enough support.

• The shoes should have good support at the arch. If you feel you need more in the arch you can add foam-rubber supports, probably available at the shoe store.

• Flexibility is an important factor in shoe selection. Bend the shoe back and forth to test pliability. The force it takes for your hand to flex the shoe will be the same force needed to flex foot muscles when you walk. Injuries can occur from too-stiff shoes.

• Laced shoes are best for proper handling and control of the foot in the shoe.

• Lightweight, ventilated nylon uppers allow air to circulate better around your feet in hot weather. Even so, leather uppers protect against rain and snow.

Break-In—Break in your new shoes by wearing them around the house for short periods of time before walking long distances. Adequate padding in the shoes can help prevent blisters. Some people wear two pairs of socks if they are prone to blistering. Socks should be absorbent and cushiony, made of wool or cotton. Be sure the socks are clean, dry and fit snugly.

Blisters and burns are produced by heat and friction. (Some people rub petroleum jelly on their feet to guard against blisters from new shoes.) If you get small blisters, don't puncture them. If you develop a large painful one, you can drain it with a sterile gauze. Don't cut the skin off the blister. Be sure you keep the area very clean and cover the blister with a sterile gauze or bandage.

With proper shoes, and by slowly increasing your mileage in your walking program, you should avoid blisters. If you have persistent muscle aches and your shoes indicate uneven wear, you may need *orthotics*. These are podiatrist-prescribed shoe inserts that redistribute weight along your foot.

GETTING READY TO WALK

My sister told me about a friend of hers who is 30 years old and overweight. They decided to play golf, but by the time they got to the third hole, her friend was exhausted. Her ankles gave out and she twisted them both. She had to stop play. I relate that episode as a warning—you may need to strengthen your ankles and feet before starting a walking program.

Walking is one of the most natural things we do. We all have our own style, doing it as unconsciously as breathing. Even so, it may seem strange that this chapter teaches people how to walk. But walking can also be very technical.

While doing research I had some frustrating times trying to understand the *biomechanics* of walking. As I walked across my living room, I tried to assimilate the terms and define each phase of the walking cycle, including the sinusoidal path of the walker, and feeling my vertical displacement within five centimeters.

I tried to master the technical equations for dealing with metabolic expenditures in slope-walking and the caloric expenditures at various speeds and grades. Radios and the TV had to be silenced so I could concentrate on the correct heel/toe angle while synchronizing my arm, leg and breathing movements. When one of my sons objected to the monastic silence, he said, "You're not going to motivate anyone to walk if you make it too complicated."

He was right! If things are too complicated, pleasure leaves and drudgery arrives. Ever since I took up running, walking had become my reward. In training and in races, I walked hills, walked when I was tired, and to rest, recover and reward myself. I love to walk, and I want you to learn to love walking too.

If you're the technical type who aspires to become an authority on the systematic study of walking, read *The Complete Book of Exercisewalking* by Gary D. Yanker. I've spent many a night curled up with a walking book and walked many a mile reading books on the subject. I'll offer you some simple tips on stride, cadence, distance, incline, breathing, posture, arm movement and foot placement. The only thing you really need to remember though, is that walking is natural and easy. Just use your common sense. You *can* do it, so please do *more* of it.

PROPER WALKING POSTURE

Keep your weight up, lift your torso and draw your breastbone up, out and forward. Your head should remain level, chin parallel to the floor. Cast your eyes four or five yards ahead.

Have your shoulders back and relaxed, buttocks tucked in firmly. Arms will swing freely in opposition to your legs. This will take just a little practice to do correctly.

When walking fast or for a long period of time, your body will tend to lean forward. Then your shoulders will rise and bunch up around the neck. Avoid this. It can cause back and neck pain plus fatigue. It will also shorten your stride.

Foot Placement—Your heel and the entire foot should be placed with toes pointed in the direction of travel, not more than two inches apart. If they are much farther apart, your body will sway from side to side in a kind of waddle.

If you walk pigeon-toed, with your toes pointed in, you will strain ankle and knee joints. A long free stride is impossible with that introverted foot position. If you are able to walk in a straight line without waddling or being pigeon-toed, your stride will be more efficient, natural and beneficial. And you'll enjoy your walk more.

Heel Placement—When walking, you should land on your heel first. This is called the *heel strike*. The heel is placed at about a 40° angle from the ground for a proper heel strike. The foot and leg are then at a 90° angle with each other. Be sure not to land flat-footed—the back edge of the heel should strike first.

Lift your foot slightly to the outside so that you will be able to roll on that side of the toe. Set your ankle slightly to the outside and that will help prevent an undesirable internal rotation of the leg. As the heel strikes, the front leg should be fully extended. When your back foot is on the ball, ready to toe-off, push straight back, not to the side.

The back leg should be fully extended at the toe-off. You should walk tall, holding your head and back erect with buttocks tucked in tightly.

ARM SWING

Swing your arms in a smooth, powerful style forward and backward just brushing your side. Bend your arms at about at 90° angle in a relaxed fist.

Synchronize your arm swing with your breathing. Inhale as you take about four to six steps, and then exhale as you take the next four to six steps. At first you may not be able to go that far on one breath until your lung capacity gradually increases.

INCREASING SPEED

When you're ready for a little more speed, the place to start is with the length of your stride. Practice reaching out with the forward-moving leg. Do this by reaching out just a few more inches than you're used to doing. You get a fuller leg extension with an erect posture, thus keeping your center of gravity higher. Speed and stride-length are related.

HOW FAST; HOW FAR?

There are several methods to determine how fast and how far you're walking. One way is to walk a measured course. Pick several nice scenic courses around your neighborhood. Drive your car along the course and measure the distance on your car's odometer. At each quarter mile, half mile, and mile make a note of a house, tree or other landmark so you will know the distance when you pass it on your walk.

On a measured course, your speed is simply a function of time and distance. To determine your speed, divide your time in minutes for a one-mile walk into 60 and you'll arrive at miles per hour.

Another way to measure mileage is by using a *pedometer* when you walk. This is a device that hooks on to your belt, pants or foot to count the number of steps you take. You adjust it to the length of your stride. Every time it feels a jolt, such as your foot striking the ground, the pedometer ticks off a unit of dis-

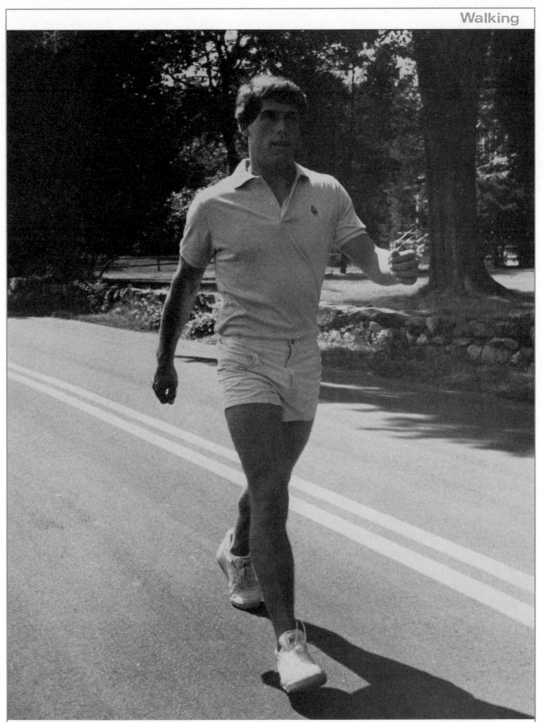

This walker is exhibiting proper technique: walking tall, good posture, vigorous arm swing, correct heel and toe placement.

tance equal to your stride. It adds them and shows you how far you've walked in miles or kilometers. However, pedometers do not work well on rough terrain that forces you to vary the length of your stride.

When you know how far you've walked, you can use the accompanying table to determine your approximate speed.

WALKING-SPEED CONVERSION TABLE

Steps Per Minute	or	Minutes Per Mile	Miles Per Hour
30		60	1.0
40		40	1.5
45		30	2.0
60		24	2.5
90		20	3.0
100		17	3.5
110		16	3.75
120		15	4.0
125		14	4.25
130		13	4.5
135		12.5	4.75
140		12	5.0
150		10.9	5.5
160		10	6.0

UP AND DOWN

There are a few techniques to keep in mind when walking stairs, hills and other inclines. The natural tendency is to go up stairs and hills on the balls of the feet, omitting the heel strike. This can make calf muscles and Achilles tendons sore. Try to walk up hills by placing your heel down first, even though it feels as if you are pressing it down. You will feel a stretch in the calf muscles.

When you descend a hill or incline, keep your posture erect, though you will have to lean backward to compensate for the sharp grade on sharp inclines.

When descending stairs, you can maintain a fully erect posture throughout. Place the heel strike down first and don't get caught in the trap of walking on the balls of your feet. You will have to walk flat-footed down stairs because you will not be able to flex your ankle as fully as on flat ground in the heel/toe roll.

ABOUT TRAFFIC

If there are no sidewalks where you are walking, face traffic and stay close to the edge of the road. Watch out for cars. If one seems to be bearing down on you, step off the road and stop walking.

When walking at night, wear a reflective vest or stripes and carry a flashlight. Get familiar with the road so you will know where there are ditches, potholes and sharp curves. If you look directly at the headlights of an oncoming car the lights can temporarily blind you so you can't see where you are going. Instead, look a little to the side.

WEATHER EXTREMES

Take special precautions in extremely hot or cold weather. In either situation, start off gradually. Always drink water before you go for a walk. When it's hot, you must drink a lot of water, so make sure your summer routes have water stops along the way. Or, carry a squeeze-bottle of water.

Test yourself in extreme weather by walking out and back within a half mile of your house. In cold weather bundle in layers. This keeps you warmer than one heavy garment. When you warm up, you can take a layer off.

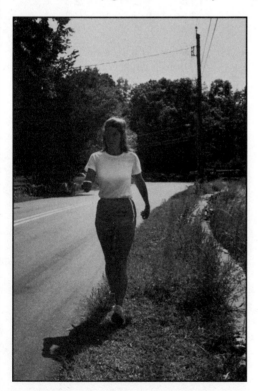

When I walk along roads, I prefer to walk at the side, against traffic. It's much safer, especially at night.

It's always colder going into the wind. Walk into the wind at the beginning of your walk so your back is to the wind when you are coming home tired and sweaty.

Indoor Walks—My father has found a remedy for walking comfortably in any weather. He walks around the indoor shopping mall in Dubuque, Iowa. The manager of the mall welcomes the walkers who cover the one-mile route

APPROXIMATE CALORIES BURNED WHILE WALKING

Food or Beverage	Portion	Calories	Minutes of Walking
Whole milk	1 cup	160	32
Ice cream	1 cup	255	51
Roast beef	3 oz.	375	75
Hamburger	3 oz.	345	49
Bacon	2 slices	60	12
Broiled chicken	3 oz.	115	23
Green beans	1/2 cup	15	3
Broccoli	1/2 cup	25	5
Celery	3 stalks	10	2
Baked potato	1	145	29
French fries	10 pieces	215	43
Apple	1 medium	80	16
Banana	1	85	17
Orange juice	1/2 cup	55	11
Whole-wheat bread	1 slice	65	13
Doughnuts	1	165	33
Spaghetti	3/4 cup	115	23
Butter or margarine	1 tbs.	100	20
Mayonnaise	1 tbs.	100	20
Chicken noodle soup	1 cup	60	13
Fudge	1 oz.	115	23
Brownie	1	90	18
Apple pie	1 piece	300	60
Pecan pie	1 piece	430	86
Cola	12 oz. can	145	29
Beer	8 oz. glass	100	20
Liquor, 86 proof	1 jigger	105	21
Table wine	1 glass	85	17
Lemonade	1/2 cup	55	11

around the corridors before the stores open. He has even offered to open the doors several hours earlier to accommodate the 75 or so walkers, many of whom are cardiac patients who could not walk otherwise unable to walk in extreme weather conditions.

My dad enjoys the friendship of the other walkers. His friend Jules, 75 years old, has lost 25 pounds by walking and controlling his diet. His blood pressure has lowered considerably and his doctor has told him he no longer needs to take his pills.

My dad and his friends have a diversion (in addition to window shopping) while they walk. They like to determine the number of minutes walking is required to burn up calories equal to those in various foods and beverages. The accompanying table equates minutes of walking with the calorie content of some common foods. The calculations are based on a 154-pound person walking at 3.5 miles per hour.

The number of calories you burn while walking varies with your speed and weight, and the inclination and ruggedness of the terrain. For example, you can burn almost twice as many calories walking in the sand as compared to walking on a hard surface. Extra calories are burned while walking when you swing your arms more, walking up an incline, or adding a weight load.

Intense activities which will burn more calories per minute can only be maintained practically by most people in 30 to 60 minutes. Jogging burns up only a few more calories per mile than fast walking. Once you have maintained a moderate level of fitness you can walk long periods of time without tiring. Walking is the best and easiest way of burning body fat. Remember, dieting alone loses lean body tissue, which will give you a saggy appearance. Lean body tissue gives you shape—you don't want to lose that.

TARGET GOALS

Begin with a measured mile. Time yourself to be sure that within a reasonable number of tries you can walk one mile in less than 15 minutes. For some people this is a brisk mile. For others it is a snap. Regardless, try to keep track of distance and time. Consider using a weekly engagement calendar to record progress.

Chapter 7 expands on this theme much more. It gives you a variety of ways to implement walking as exercise. In addition, it describes how you can walk, bike and swim your way to good health.

SUMMARY

Now you have my secrets to fitness success through walking: Get the correct walking shoes. Walk as I have directed. Continue to lengthen your strides. And increase mileage and decrease time within your individual capabilities.

CHAPTER FIVE

Bicycling

I got my first bike for my 7th birthday. As a 10-year-old tomboy I raced up and down sidewalks, riding "no-hands." Then, between the ages of 13 and 40 I was on a bike no more than five times.

HUMBLE BEGINNINGS

My motives for returning to biking had to do with energy conservation and physical fitness. At the time, there was a gas shortage with hour-long lines at gas stations. On top of that, I was experiencing a money shortage. My three kids and I were all enrolled in college and none of us were about to forego an education for that gas-guzzling, rusting wreck on wheels, my car.

A bicycle was the answer to my transportation problems! So I hopped on my son's bike and rode one block to disaster. I ended up sprawled on the grass with the bike on top of me, wondering if I had broken any bones or had a heart attack from fear.

What happened was that I instinctively pushed back on the pedals to slow down on the hill. When my son realized what was happening, he shouted after me, "The brakes are on the handlebars!" I grabbed the brakes and squeezed them as hard as I could. The bike stopped abruptly, but I kept going—and the first of many bicycle lectures followed. My son found fault with me for starting out on a hill, getting on a bike that was too big for me, not knowing my equipment, and more.

The next week at a garage sale I found the perfect bike. It was just like the one I rode 30 years before, and it cost only $8. I pedaled around town feeling like a kid again. My daughter was a little embarrassed to have me riding an old-fashioned bike with balloon tires and upright handlebars. But I ignored her and rode every day for a week—until I was hit by a car.

I saw the car coming out of the intersection. The driver was looking the other way for traffic as he slowly pulled out. I jumped off the bike the second before he smashed into it. The driver got out of his car and shouted at me for being dumb enough to ride on the wrong side of the street. (He was right.)

He extracted my crumpled bike from his fender and threw it in the weeds near where I was sitting and drove off. I just sat there and cried. Finally I stumbled home and announced to my family that I was an old woman, that I was going to quit school, give up sports and submerge myself in soap operas.

Solution—A few days later, my kids got me to reconsider. They presented me with a new 12-speed bike and a triathlon application, filled out and waiting for my signature. The boys told me they would coach me. My daughter described an image of me training with other athletes and entering triathlons.

I have learned a lot since then through mistakes, study and experience. I want to share my experience with you—not so you'll become an Ironman—but so you too can know the exhilaration of safe cycling to good health. Cycling has become my favorite sport, and I hope it will also become yours.

BIKING BENEFITS

There are no age, weight or height restrictions for bicycling. It is a complete form of exercise that benefits arms, shoulders, back, diaphragm and legs. Your mind can free itself of stress as you relax and experience the carefree feeling created by rhythmic pedaling. Feel the wind on your face, sense your environment, watch how the changing scenery lifts your spirit. I love to watch the birds while I'm biking. I feel as though I'm flying right along with them.

A 1980 survey showed that more than 90 million bicycles were owned by Americans, an increase of 70 million in a 20-year period. Cycling is now ranked as the fourth most popular sport in the United States.

Other Reasons to Bicycle—In addition to this popular recreational use of bicycles, many people also use their bicycles for commuting and running errands. Studies show that more than half the trips made in cars are short trips, five miles or less. It is estimated that if bicycles were used for these trips, families could save close to $1,000 a year in fuel costs. The amount of gasoline used for transportation in the United States would drop significantly and this would also have an impact on air quality in many places.

Cycling offers the versatility of riding with family, friends, bicycle clubs or alone.

CHOOSING YOUR BICYCLE

Because there are so many types of cycling and kinds of bicycles, I'm going to review them first. Then you'll learn how you can best incorporate a bicycle into your low-stress fitness routine.

Selecting the right bicycle is a very personal decision but I can offer some advice from research and experience. Perhaps you already have a bicycle sitting idly in the garage, or you feel you have no desire to bicycle. All I ask is that you keep an open mind as you read this chapter.

When I describe various types of cycling exercise, take a few minutes to picture yourself in those circumstances. When you're out of shape and not feeling very good about yourself, it's hard to think of exercise as fun. I can almost guarantee that if you enter your exercise program slowly, correctly and with a positive attitude, these will become "lifesports." Think of investment in a bicycle as an investment in physical and mental health.

FINANCIAL CONSIDERATIONS

I started out riding an $8 clunker. Now I ride a $1,500 custom, racing bike. It would have been a mistake for me to start out on the expensive bike even if I had the money. I would have soon wrecked it because I didn't know the rules of the road; I had terrible fears; and I had a mental block about shifting gears. You, on the other hand, are going about it sensibly by reading a book that instructs you in basic techniques.

Used Bike—If money, or lack of it, is a prime consideration in buying a bicycle, I suggest starting with a good, used bicycle. With a basic understanding of the bicycle and its components, you can make a wise purchase.

Cyclists often *trade up* or buy better bikes as they become more involved in the sport. Consequently, well-maintained bikes can be purchased from these people or from shops that sell used bikes.

If you are a bike novice, I highly recommend that you purchase a bicycle from a *reputable bicycle dealer.* There should be a wide selection of bikes that have been correctly assembled. Typically, you will be able to test-ride it after the shop owner adjusts it to fit your body.

Also, if you have any problems with the bike once you purchase it, or need replacement parts, a reputable store will guarantee and service it.

Discount Bikes—At a discount store, bikes are rarely sold assembled. A bicycle dealer once told me that people often bring discount bikes to him to be assembled. He charges $30! The total spent on a "discount" bike plus assembly charges can typically buy a better quality, assembled bicycle from a dealer who would also back the bicycle and service it.

THE 10-SPEED BICYCLE

The bicycle I rode in my first year of competition was a 12-speed, discount-store special. It had a flashy paint job and was very heavy. I trained on it for three months before my first triathlon. I rode down hills with my brakes on, rarely changed gears, and rode so close to curbs that I usually scraped the pedals.

It was the night before my first triathlon that a fellow competitor showed me how to operate the gears in a way that made sense. A well-meaning cyclist had given me a gear-ratio chart that would have taken a math major to decipher. So, before you venture into the cyclist's domain or out onto the road, acquaint yourself with a few of the basics.

In my opinion, the most versatile type of bicycle is a good, 10-speed *sport-touring bicycle.* Most "10-speeds" feature straight-frame tubing, two-derailleur gearing, narrow rims and tires, dropped handlebars and a racing-style saddle. These bikes are priced from $200 on up. Generally, the better the bike, the more expensive it will be.

A good 10-speed is versatile enough for recreational riding, commuting, racing or for a touring vacation. Even so, there *are* high-quality, specialty bikes designed for each of those endeavors. But I'm taking the generalist's approach for now, assuming that you are a relative newcomer to biking. I want you to invest in a bicycle that will give you years of fitness and pleasure.

Dropped Handlebar—You might not like a 10-speed because you think dropped handlebars are uncomfortable and will cause back problems. Actually, the reverse is true. With *correctly adjusted,* dropped handlebars, you can ride in at least five different positions. By changing positions you can relieve any stress on arms, shoulders and hands. Conventional, flat handlebars offer only one or two positions.

When riding with dropped handlebars with hands on top, your back is at about a 45° angle. In this position spinal segments are much farther apart than when you sit upright. This makes road shock better absorbed by both spine and arms.

Your spine is more compressed in the upright position. Arms cannot absorb much body weight. Road shock is then transferred to your body.

A little guidance and practice will get you used to dropped handlebars. But they must be correctly adjusted—more on that later.

Bicycle Seats—A comfortable seat, or *saddle,* is important. The narrow style typically found on 10-speeds is designed to prevent chafing by supporting your pelvis and allowing your legs to move freely. When the bike is correctly adjusted to you, body weight rests on both the seat and handlebars—not *just* the seat. Also, much of your weight is distributed to the pedals when riding. This way, comfort comes not just from the softness of the saddle but also from the way the adjusted bike accommodates your body.

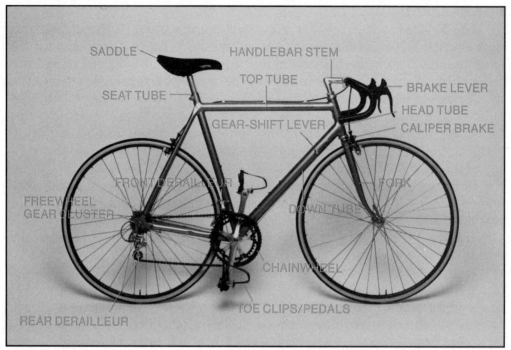

These are the basic parts of a 10-speed bike. Photo courtesy of Cannondale.

Avoid saddles that are wide and heavy. You don't want your thighs to scrape the saddle. This causes painful chafing and wastes leg energy. Also avoid saddles with spring "shocks." They will inhibit transfer of force to the pedals.

Most bicycles in the low- to medium-price ranges come with molded plastic saddles that are uncomfortable for anything but short rides. If you find that your bicycle seat is particularly uncomfortable, purchase a new one. You can get a super seat for about $25. Only experienced bikers should consider getting a hard-leather seat or one with glove leather on a plastic frame. Most people will prefer a saddle with compressed (not spongy) padding in the rear. It offers a pleasant compromise between comfort and efficiency.

Because of anatomical differences, women should buy special saddles. These are wider in the back part of the seat because women have different pelvic bone structure. Conventional saddles are too narrow to offer comfortable support. Typically, well-designed saddles are available in both male and female models.

ALL-TERRAIN BIKE

The so-called *mountain bike,* or all-terrain bike, is a relative newcomer that is rapidly gaining popularity. It has a strong, touring-bike frame and wide wheels with knobby tires. Tires are sturdy, resist punctures and have better traction on muddy, grassy, or gravel surfaces. These bikes have straight, reinforced handlebars, and saddles are typically wider than those found on 10-speeds.

Mountain bikes usually come with 15 to 18 speeds, which makes hill climbing easy. They are relatively maintenance-free because they are designed for rough conditions and have fewer flats than other types of bikes.

All-terrain bikes offer a fine alternative to the 10-speed design. They will go just about anywhere and can carry quite a load. They are usually more expensive than the same quality 10-speed bike.

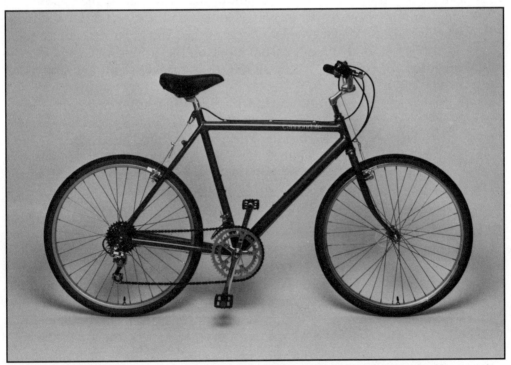

For "go-anywhere" urban or country riding, I suggest that you look into getting a mountain bike, such as this Cannondale model. It has most of the features of a conventional 10-speed, but has wider tires, a sturdier frame and upright handlebars.

ONE- AND THREE-SPEED BICYCLES

Good one-speed and three-speed bicycles are also available. They are designed for longevity and short rides, not for speed or performance. This tends to make them heavier than 10-speed or all-terrain bikes. One-speed bikes typically have coaster brakes. *Some* three-speed bikes have hand brakes.

If you live in an area with level terrain and plan to use your bicycle only occasionally for exercise, you may prefer either type. But I think that as you become more involved in cycling and experience the pleasure it can bring, you may wish you had a bicycle with more performance capabilities.

ADULT TRICYCLES

There's no performance from an adult "trike," but they allow a lot of people to bicycle who otherwise couldn't at all. Use one if it is *the only way* you can bicycle. Adult bicycles are good for people with balance problems, but there are some maneuvering considerations to take into account. In fact, adult tricycles can be dangerous if you are not aware of this.

The problem is in turning. When turning at slow or moderate speeds, you must lean slightly *away* from the direction of the turn. This is the opposite of what you do on a two-wheeler, leaning slightly *into* the direction of the turn. Practice in a vacant parking lot to get the feel of this. You must shift your weight to the outer rear wheel to prevent it from lifting off the ground.

Remember: On a tricycle you lean left while turning right; and lean right while turning left.

Another thing to be careful about with trikes is that when you ride on a sidewalk over a driveway, it tends to turn in the direction of the slope, toward the street. You simply have to force the wheel back so you'll go straight.

In my research I've found that the Schwinn three-wheeler is excellent among domestic models. It corners well, with with less tendency for the wheel to lift than some other brands.

EXERCISE BICYCLES

Exercise bicycles for indoor "riding" are available in a variety of models and price ranges. For example, Schwinn produces an Air-Dyne Ergo Metric exercise bicycle that sells for over $400. One nice feature it and other models offer is *progressive resistance* so you can adjust the ease of pedaling. Some models also feature handlebar action. In addition to pedaling, you can pump handlebars with both arms. This lets you work the upper body along with the lower body.

Whether you bicycle indoors or outdoors, you use essentially the same muscles. If you live in a climate with inclement weather, an exercise bicycle might be for you.

But I prefer the best of both worlds, so I use my bike on a device called a *wind-load trainer.* It turns my racing bike into a stationary bicycle. I remove the front wheel and mount the bike on the stand. The back wheel rests on two small turbine-type blower wheels. The spinning turbines create a drag effect that imitates wind resistance. It enables me to shift gears to vary my workouts. And I get to work out on a bike that already has been adjusted for my body.

The problem with an *ordinary* stationary bicycle is that you can't go for a ride outside on nice days. That's the real joy of cycling. My training stand permits me to adapt my cycling to the weather.

PROPER FIT AND ADJUSTMENTS

In my opinion, too many people learned to dislike bicycling while using incorrectly sized or adjusted machines. Indeed, the wrong bike *is* uncomfortable and dangerous.

Following are general recommendations in getting the right fit for pleasant and safe biking. Some are hard to actually do and evaluate yourself. You'll need a friend if you are adjusting an old bike. If you are buying a new or used bike from a reputable dealer, have a shop person help you adjust the bike.

FRAME SIZE

Once you decide which *type* bicycle you want, you need to determine appropriate frame size. You can adjust the seat and handlebars for a comfortable and efficient ride, but the basic frame size cannot be changed. A frame that is too large is a hazard in mounting, dismounting and stopping, so you must start out with the correct size. For adults, the right frame size won't change.

Ideally, when you straddle a bike with both feet on the ground, there should be one to two inches clearance between the top bar and your crotch. The key measurement for determining the frame size for you is your *inseam,* the distance between the floor and crotch. Make this measurement in your bare feet.

Ads often describe bikes as a *26-inch man's bike* or a *24-inch girl's bike.* This usually refers to the *diameter of the wheel,* which is different from *frame size.* Most adult 10-speeds use a 27-inch wheel, regardless of frame size. Other types of bikes use other standards. The illustration on page 120 will help familiarize you with terminology of some bicycle parts.

SEAT POSITION

First, get a friend to help you with these adjustments. If necessary, go to a bike store and get expert help.

Saddle Height—Have someone hold the bicycle upright while you are seated on it with barefeet. Center a heel on a pedal in the 6:00 position and straighten that leg. If the saddle adjustment is correct, your leg should be just fully

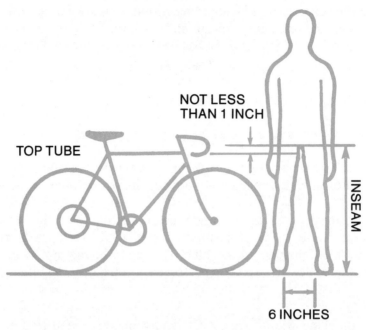

Another way to determine proper frame size is to choose a frame with a top bar that is about one inch below your crotch, if you stand as shown.

FRAME SIZE vs. INSEAM

Frame Size	Inseam
17"	26" to 30"
19"	28" to 31"
20"	29" to 32"
21"	30" to 33"
22"	31" to 34"
23"	32" to 35"
24"	33" to 36"
25"	34" to 37"
26"	35" to 38"

To measure frame size, use a tape measure to measure the distance between the top of the frame's seat tube and the center of the front chain ring. In this way *frame size* is the same as *seat-tube length*. A 19-inch frame will have a 19-inch seat tube.

extended. You may have to move the seat up and down to find the correct height. When you find the right position, adjust the tightening device with the appropriate wrench.

Seat height is important because if the seat is too low, leg muscles never fully stretch and are always tensed. This leads to premature fatigue or cramping. If you notice someone bouncing in the saddle with each leg stroke, the seat is probably too low.

A saddle that is too high can cause pain in the crotch and soreness in the legs. Also you will not have fluid of leg movements when your leg muscles are stretched beyond maximum capacity. If you notice someone's hips rocking left and right with each leg stroke, the saddle is probably too high.

Correct frame size is important to correct saddle height because there should be at least 2-1/2 inches of the seat post inside the frame's seat tube. If not, the seat and post won't stay adjusted. Worse, it might break off from stress or metal fatigue.

There should be a little post showing. If the saddle is right against the seat tube, the frame is too large.

Saddle Angle—Adjust it so it's about level from front to back. Determine this by placing a yardstick on the saddle, making the straight edge parallel with the top tube of the frame. There is some controversy over whether the saddle should be straight or actually tipped up from the front end. If the level position is not comfortable, make tiny adjustments in the up direction and experiment to find what is best for you. But before making changes, ride for several hours first.

Saddle's Horizontal Distance—The correct forward/backward adjustment of the saddle position is designed to accommodate differences in thigh length and riding styles. The correct setting insures the right angle of leg thrust.

Generally, the nose of the saddle should be 2 to 2-1/2 inches behind the centerline of the *bottom bracket*—the housing of the bearing mechanism in the center of the whole pedal assembly. Determine this by dropping a plumb line from the saddle nose and adjust the saddle appropriately.

HANDLEBARS

Handlebar height is usually from about saddle height to three inches below, depending on personal comfort.

The horizontal extension of dropped handlebars is a bit more complicated: Sit on the correctly adjusted seat with hands on the top of the handlebars, which are at the right height. A plumb line (imaginary or real) dropped from your nose should be about an inch behind the front of the handlebars.

Also, dropped handlebars should be as wide as the rider's shoulders.

I recommend *sponge handlebar covers* to add comfort. Ordinarily handlebars are wrapped with cotton or canvas tape, which does nothing to soften the surface. Bicycle shops carry cushioned handlebar covers that are well worth the price.

BRAKES

Brake levers on handlebars need to be within easy reach and work properly. Before you buy or ride a bike, test the brakes by squeezing the brake levers hard. There should be less than an inch of motion before the brakes act. They should not go all the way to the handlebars.

If they do, they either aren't adjusted properly because there is too much cable slack, or the brakes themselves will distort and bend. Check the front and back brake separately. Stand next to the bike, firmly apply the front brake and try to push the bike forward. The front wheel should not move. Test the back brake in the same way.

Brake *extension levers* are horizontal levers attached to the main levers on dropped handlebars. They allow you to brake with the hands on the top of the bar. This may seem more convenient, but braking action is not enhanced any. Many cycling authorities eschew them, recommending that you remove them from any bike that has them.

If you become used to these levers, you may not be able to stop in time in an emergency. If you have small, weak hands, don't be concerned about operating hand brakes with the main levers. With practice, it will become second nature.

Never ride a bicycle if the brakes are not working properly. A bicycle shop can replace or adjust them if you can't do it yourself.

TOE CLIPS

Toe clips are cage-like devices on pedals. They are designed to increase the efficiency of power transfer between foot and pedal. Essentially, you can power the bike with both down- and upstroke, increasing efficiency from 35% to 45%.

Even so, many people don't like them because they feel partly "trapped" in the bike. That's valid if the clips aren't adjusted properly or if you aren't an experienced rider. City riding especially can be hazardous if the clips are too tight. It does take a while to get used to them, but in the long run you will benefit from using them.

A few types of toe clips are available. "Old-style" designs use curved-metal clips and leather straps. Newer designs include clips made of curved-metal only. Straps aren't necessary. This type may be for you because the design lets your foot feel "freer."

What I Did—During the several months I rode to reacquaint myself with bicycling, I accustomed myself first to dropped handlebars, hand brakes and the top-bar position before I tried to use toe clips. After practicing inserting and removing my feet from the clips, I practiced riding with the straps a bit tighter. When I felt secure in bending down to release the straps for stops, I purchased bicycle shoes with built-in toe clips. (These are necessary for racing only.)

It took me several months and a few falls before I felt comfortable being strapped securely on the pedals for racing. I'm glad I persisted because mastering the toe clips has improved my cycling as well as boosted my ego by overcoming the challenge.

HELMETS, REFLECTORS AND LIGHTS

All cyclists should wear modern helmets designed for bicyclists. The only time I pedal without one is when I'm on my stationary bike. Buy a bicycle helmet and get in the habit of wearing it even for very short rides.

Aside from the obvious protection it offers your head in the event of a fall, I find a psychological benefit. It's a reminder to "use my head," to be alert and cautious. I have developed quicker reflexes as a result of bicycling. For example, I noticed great improvements in my tennis game after a year of cycling. I was able to keep my eye on the ball, concentrate and relax. These things I did not do well before bicycling.

If your habit is to ride when it's dark—something I don't recommend—your bike *must* be equipped with lights and reflectors. Safety and legal resons demand it. In some states you can't buy a new bike that does not come equipped with reflectors. And you could be ticketed by the police for not using a light at night. Check with your local bike store for appropriate reflectors and lights.

CYCLING CLOTHES

"Official" bicycle clothes will not only add to the comfort of your ride but will also distinguish you as a cyclist. I felt a bit silly the first time I wore cycling clothes because they look so different, but now I always wear them. Due to the popularity of bicycling, a huge variety of cycling clothes is available. You can find exciting colors, cuts, fabrics and designs to fit just about any need.

Shorts—Cycling shorts are tight-fitting, made of a material such as acrylic, wool, Spandex or various blends that provide unrestricted motion. Racing-style shorts are made long and smooth with special seams so you avoid chafing as your legs rub against the saddle. A piece of chamois or other soft material is typically sewn into the crotch for padding and to prevent chafing from any inside seams.

Touring-style shorts are a bit different because they may have pockets and

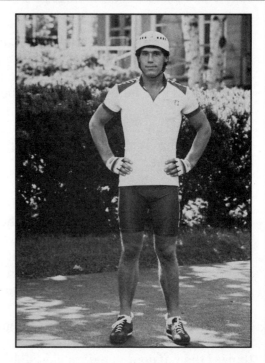

Appropriate bicycling clothes definitely help you ride long distances better. They make excellent gifts to yourself or others because they can provide years of protection and comfort. In giving gifts of athletic gear you're helping to promote fitness.

a different cut for general use too. Most shorts of both styles have elastic waists and are cut low in the front for easier breathing and higher in the back to keep your lower back covered as you lean forward.

Shirts—Traditional *bicycle jerseys* are cut longer and fit tighter than regular shirts. The reason for the tight fit is to reduce wind resistance. They usually have large pockets across the back for carrying food, maps or personal items.

Skin Suits—These one-piece suits are currently very popular. They fit tight and offer the benefits of the aforementioned shorts and shirts.

My daughter always borrows mine, saying she rides better when she is dressed like a cyclist. I found this to be true in most sports. If you dress the part, your performance usually improves. That's why I like to encourage people to acquire athletic outfits designed for their sport, even if they are novices. It gives a little extra incentive to stay with the sport and assures added comfort, especially in the case of cycling shorts. Styles of active sportswear tend to stay "in style" for a long time, giving you many years of wear.

Gloves—Bicycling gloves have padded palms and half fingers. The back is usually mesh, fitted with Velcro closures at the wrist. These gloves will add to your comfort as you support your body weight and absorb shock while you lean on the handlebars. They are also a safety device if you are so unfortunate as to fall and skid on your hands. For this reason alone, many people wear bicycling gloves.

Shoes—Cycling shoes come in two styles, the traditional racing design with *cleats,* and touring shoes. The purpose of a cycling shoe is to keep your feet from flexing while transmitting power to the pedal. They are designed with thin, rigid soles, are cut narrow for easy use in toe clips, and are often ventilated for coolness.

The cleats of racing shoes fit into special pedals that make the rider's foot connect to the pedal. This better enables the rider to pull up on the pedals as well as push down for greater riding efficiency.

I don't recommend these unless speed and performance are very important to you. In addition, cleated shoes make walking very difficult.

I recommend a *touring shoe.* They are are usually less expensive and are easier to walk in than racing designs. Most touring models have stiff reinforced soles that are molded with inset grooves that act as cleats to hold your feet straight on the pedal.

Soft-soled shoes such as tennis or running shoes are not recommended for cycling more than a few miles. For long distances you need a stiffer sole to protect your feet.

ACCESSORY EQUIPMENT

Bicycles should be outfitted with a few accessories for safety and convenience. For some people, these are essentials, not accessories. Basically, the difference depends on your level of involvement and distances you travel.

Water Bottle—A water bottle that attaches to your bike is important if you're riding more than a couple miles, especially in hot weather. Cyclists need to be aware of the dangers of dehydration. Its first symptom is lack of perspiration. The breeze of riding tends to fool riders into thinking that sweat is just evaporating quickly. But that's not necessarily true. Drink water often.

Bags and Racks—Bicycle shops also carry a variety of *bags* and *racks* that can be fitted to your bike. A small bag attached under their saddle can easily hold a spare tire, tools, patch kit, rag, bicycle lock, personal identification and some money. All of these things have proved necessary for me at various times.

One of the beauties of cycling is the feeling of independence and the ability to cover miles rather quickly. In the event of a flat you don't want to be miles from home and stranded. Changing a bicycle tire is really not that difficult. It's a good idea to learn at home by deflating your tire and practicing changing it. Or, take a bike-repair class at a local bike store. Then, when you need to fix something on the road, you won't be too inconvenienced.

Pump—A tire pump is another piece of equipment you will need. Pumps come in two basic styles. One type fits on the frame and goes where you go. The other is a stand-up type that doesn't travel with you, but is easier to use. I have both kinds. Because I may travel far, I like the security of having a pump with me.

In fact, the end of the pump that attaches to the tire valve comes in two styles because tire valves do too. *Presta* valves are the skinny ones; *Schrader* valves are the thick ones similar to the valves on auto tires.

A *pressure gauge,* which is about the size of a pencil and costs a few dollars, helps you monitor tire pressure. Correct tire pressure provides longer tire life in addition to a safer and more efficient ride. Too much pressure may overstress the tire, blow it off the rim, or increase the chance of puncture from small objects. It is not a good idea to inflate your tires with gas-station air pumps. The powerful pump inflates your tire too rapidly. This can cause problems, as the tire might stretch excessively at one point before the entire tube fills.

HOW TO RIDE A BIKE

If you have never ridden a bicycle or if you have not been on one for a number of years, ask an experienced friend to help you start. Have him stand in front of the handlebars facing you with the front wheel wedged between his legs. He should hold the handlebars firmly to keep the bicycle upright. Sit on the bike and practice balancing and leaning.

Riding a bicycle is primarily a matter of mastering balance while you are on the bike and traveling straight. With your friend holding the bike, lean to the left and then to the right. As your bicycle leans to one side, practice leaning to the opposite side just enough to counteract the forces which would make the bike fall. The bike leans one way, you lean the other.

The shifts in leaning or balance you need to make to stay up are very small. Typically, they are about an inch or two one way or the other. Practice that awhile until you react automatically and feel secure.

OUTDOOR PRACTICE

Try riding your bicycle outside now. In spite of what I said earlier, lower the seat far enough so when you sit on it both feet can be firmly planted on the ground. With both hands on the handlebars, push the bike along with your feet in a scootering motion. You will soon realize that you can push and raise your feet to travel several yards, balancing and steering all the time.

If you are on a slight downgrade, you won't have to scoot. Practice moving your hands to different positions on the handlebars and cautiously use the brakes.

Now raise your seat back up to the right position and then ask a friend (one in good shape!) to run alongside you when you ride. The friend should give you moral and physical support by encouraging you to stay relaxed and catch you if you start to fall.

Turns—Corners take practice, so start out on deserted streets or empty parking lots before riding in traffic. When you make right-angle turns, you must be able to negotiate them without taking them too wide and swerving into the line of traffic.

If you are going too fast when approaching a corner, brake slowly *before* you turn. Do not apply brakes *as* you turn. If you don't brake evenly, you could lose control and fall. Always be alert for traffic.

Braking—Get into the habit of testing your brakes before each ride. I had the terrifying experience of realizing halfway down a hill that my quick-release brakes were not engaged correctly.

Be sure to practice *panic stops* so you can react instantly when the situation arises. Panic stops are needed when a car door opens suddenly in front of you, or when an animal or person darts into your path.

To make such an emergency stop, bend down and extend your bottom as far back on the saddle as you can. At the same time, squeeze the brake levers hard. Pushing your weight over the rear wheel will help distribute weight evenly and keep the braked wheels from skidding.

Try not to let your speed build when you go down a hill. Hard braking at high speeds builds up *friction heat*. This could cause a blowout and be very dangerous, especially at high speeds. To avoid heat buildup on a steep hill, use *alternate braking*. Apply the rear brake for a moment, then use the front brake while the rear one cools. Repeat this until you are down the hill.

RIDING SAFELY

You can practice steering straight by following lines painted on the road edge. Try to stay a constant distance from the side of the road. Be alert for potholes, sticks, glass, wet leaves, sand and gravel on the side of the road. Avoid running over them.

Grated storm-sewer covers pose a real hazard too. They are dangerous to ride over and tough on your tires. Also be cautious when crossing railroad or streetcar tracks. You should cross them at a right angle at slow speed. Some bikers prefer to walk their bikes across.

Dogs cause a problem when they come barking after you. They usually are protecting their territory, so the sooner you get away the better. Bike away as fast as you can. If you can safely reach your water bottle without slowing down, give them a good squirt in the face.

About Traffic Regulations—Don't forget that you must obey all local driving regulations—from stop signs to signalling turns. (But don't worry about maintaining the speed limit.) Observe all traffic regulations.

- Always ride with the traffic (stay to the right), never into it—that's why I was hit by a car. I thought I would be safer seeing the cars coming toward me. Had the police come, I would have been cited for being on the wrong side of the road.

- You will probably be a little nervous at first when traffic is going by you. If you don't get used to it, stay on the emptiest roads you can find or push for local bike paths in your community.

- Make sure that motorists can see you. Wear brightly colored clothing.

- If you cycle in the dark, use reflectors on your bike or clothes and use a light for the front and back. Reflectors should be on all sides—especially the wheels and pedals—because drivers identify them as belonging to a cyclist.

- Use *hand signals* to indicate turning and stopping. Your signals to motorists, pedestrians and other cyclists should be clear, definite and accurate.

Point the way you want to go. I've avoided a lot of accidents that way. I have had several close calls on bicycle paths where children were cycling toward me. It's too confusing to say, "Stay right" or "Stay left." Instead, determine the safest side for them to pass, point to where you want them to be and in a commanding voice say, "Stay on this side."

- Ride *defensively* and intelligently for safe and enjoyable rides. When I am at a stop sign and not sure if the car next to me is going to turn right, I'll tap on the window to get the driver's attention and motion the direction I'm going. Know ahead of time how a cyclist would handle traffic situations, and you'll avoid being frightened and insecure before something happens.

- A left-hand turn with traffic around you can be harrowing if you don't know how to execute it safely. The safest method is to cross the street, stop, wait for the light to change, then walk across the other street with the pedestrians. Children and beginning cyclists should make left-hand turns this way.

- *Never* try to make a left-hand turn from the right curb position. Signal traffic behind you, making certain they see you. Move to the center of the road as you approach the intersection. Signal your intentions and make the left turn when you can do it safely.

- When I start up from a traffic light, I like to cross the intersection with a car to my left. It "runs interference" for me. Be careful of buses. Don't ride beside them—especially to their right—because they have to frequently pull over to the curb to let passengers off.

- Stay off turnpikes and freeways. It is definitely dangerous and illegal.
- In some cities, it is best to avoid streets where parking is not allowed. Where parking is prohibited, there is typically no room for you between the traffic and curb. These streets have a high volume of traffic. Cars could force you into the curb.

Where cars are allowed to park, there have to be three feet between moving traffic and parked cars. Unless you're a beginner cyclist, that should allow you enough room.

- When riding past parked cars, get in the habit of keeping an eye out for occupants who might open a door suddenly. Whistle or shout to make your presence known.
- Pedestrians have the right of way at all intersections, as do cars on your right. I give everybody the right of way when I'm cycling. Then I feel safe and relaxed.
- When cycling in a group, ride single file and warn the riders behind you of obstacles in the road. Use hand signals to inform those behind you before you turn or stop.
- Obey all stoplights, stop signs and other road signs, but don't assume other drivers will stop. Again, *ride defensively.*
- Never wear headphones to listen to music because the music will block out traffic noise and you won't be able to hear approaching cars or bikes. I have often been tempted to listen to music when taking four-hour rides, but I change my mind because it's much too dangerous. Many states prohibit wearing headphones while cycling or running on the streets.

PROPER RIDING TECHNIQUE

Do not mount your bicycle by putting one foot on a pedal and throwing your other leg over the bike cowboy fashion. Rather, straddle the top tube before placing your foot on a pedal. With one foot squarely on the pavement, place the opposite foot on a pedal that is at 45° above the ground.

Check for traffic, then push off with the foot on the ground while lifting your weight on to the 45° pedal. Then place the pushing foot on the pedal and lift yourself onto the saddle. This gives *full starting power* for adequate speed and maximum control.

To dismount, carefully apply the brakes and support your weight on the downside pedal. Then pull your body forward from the saddle and step to the ground with your opposite foot, bringing the bicycle to a stop. Practice getting on and off the bike, turning, balancing and braking. Become comfortable and secure before you concern yourself with the gears.

ABOUT GEARING

If you have a 5- or 10-speed bike, don't be intimidated by the gears. They are not very hard to understand. This advice comes to you from one who had "gear fear for a year." Remember, I challenged myself to compete in a triathlon in spite of the bicycling fear caused by my accident. By pressuring myself, I had developed a mental block about gears.

That's why I keep telling you to make your exercise and cycling a relaxed playtime. A relaxed mind and body will have improved concentration and coordination. My son patiently explained to me over and over how to operate the gears and change bike tires. It puzzled me that I just wasn't able to comprehend and feel at ease with those aspects of cycling.

The solution finally came one day when I was trying to reattach my back tire. I was covered with grease and he said to me, "Mom, this is the tenth time I've told you how to do this." I lashed back at him, "I'm a mother, not a mechanic! Women should not have to do this!" It was then that I realized I had been subconsciously rejecting mechanical abilities because I thought they were unfeminine.

Read through this section on gearing. When you're relaxed, experiment with your bike on a quiet, level street. I wish I had been able to learn it this way.

The Beginning—A 10-speed bicycle will provide a pleasurable ride because you can adjust the gearing to fit terrain and wind conditions. You change gears with *shift levers* on the handlebars or on the diagonal tube of the frame. There are two shift mechanisms on a 10-speed bike, each operated by a separate shift lever.

Typically the left lever moves the *front derailleur.* It moves the chain to different *chain rings,* or *front gears.* The other lever operates the *rear derailleur.* It moves the chain along the collection of five small sprockets called the *freewheel cluster.*

On a 10-speed the chain can be in five different positions for both front chain rings. That's where the 10 speeds come from. An 18-speed bike has three front chain rings and a freewheel cluster with 6 sprockets. More speeds mean a wider range of gearing from easy to difficult.

Start Shifting—Have someone hold the bike so the rear wheel is off the ground while you operate and observe gear changes. Until you become accustomed to shifting to all speeds, it is easier to operate just the rear derailleur. When you have mastered the rear gears, you can begin to use the front ones.

Twirl the pedals while you are changing the gears. When riding you *must* always be pedaling as you shift the gears. With the pedals moving, push the right-side shift lever all the way forward. This moves the chain to the smallest rear sprocket. If the chain also is on the large front chain ring, you are in *the highest speed gear*—number 10 on a 10-speed bike.

This is the hardest speed to pedal in, but you move farthest with each revolution. You use this gear for downhill, or on level ground only after you have warmed up and are moving well. Do not use this high gear in the beginning because you will tire too quickly and might hurt your knees. Do not use bicycling as a form of weight training by pushing difficult gears. By using the correct speeds, you will become a strong cyclist who can ride for hours without tiring.

Now shift the gears again with the pedals moving. When you pull the right shift lever toward you, the rear derailleur moves the chain to the largest of the rear sprockets.

You have shifted to an easier-to-pedal gear. It might help when you start riding to tape a reminder to this effect on your handlebars. It could read, *Gear lever near is easy; Far is hard.* This is true only for the right lever or rear gear.

Now experiment with the left shift lever to see what the front derailleur does. See if pulling the lever toward you puts the chain on the large or small front chain ring. I have two 10-speeds, and the left gear levers operate differently on each.

Just remember this: The right shift lever operates the rear derailleur. When the chain is on the smallest rear cog that's high gear, and it's harder to pump. The left lever operates the front derailleur. When the chain is on the smallest front cog, it's the lowest gear.

Selecting Gears—For the purposes of this book, you don't have to learn everything about which gears to use. What's good for one person may not necessarily be right for another. Basically, you want to be in a gear that is *comfortable to maintain.* If the gear is too high, your legs will get too tired. If it's too low, you will run out of breath. Generally, it's better to err on the easy side than strain yourself pushing hard gears.

You must always be pedaling forward, not backward, while you are shifting gears. Move the shift lever *firmly* but do not force it. When shifting up or down, the sequence is to shift one rear gear first, then shift the front gear if necessary. When you need the next gear, change the gear at the rear. Think of the front gear as a *halfway gear* between each of the rear cogs.

On Hills—Shift to select an easier gear *as you approach* a steep hill. If you wait until you are halfway up, the strain on the mechanisms will inhibit the derailleur from shifting. The chain has to be moving to effect a shift, but it cannot be transmitting power.

If you find yourself on a hill that is too steep to execute a gear change, and you are slowing down, release your toe clips and get off the bike. Several times this happened to me, but I waited too long before I got off the bike. The result was a slow-motion fall. At that point all you can do is a lot of cursing before you hit the ground.

When Stopping—Shift into low gear before coming to a complete stop. This way, when you start you'll be in an appropriately low gear.

Noises—Get in the habit of listening to the chain as you shift. A *rattling sound* after you shift usually means the chain has not set properly on the sprockets. Gently adjust the shift lever until the noise stops.

A *scraping noise* indicates a derailleur is not in the right position, causing the chain to rub against it. Adjust the shift levers to eliminate the noise, or the derailleur may be affected.

Using Friends—Don't shy away from 10-speed bikes or be overwhelmed by the complexity of the gears. With a little patience and practice, you will master them. When I was struggling to learn the gears, I found it helpful to have a cyclist friend along to point out the appropriate gears as we rode over different terrains.

PEDALING

Cadence is the number of revolutions per minute (RPM) that you turn the pedals. Our aim in cycling is to be able to maintain a constant high number of RPMs without wearing out. This is generally accomplished by pedaling rapidly in low gears. Cyclists call this *spinning*. Once you have mastered the art of spinning you will be able to travel long distances without tiring. You change your gears according to terrain and wind conditions to maintain this cadence.

The average rider usually pedals less than 40 RPMs. An accomplished cyclist will have a cadence between 60 and 90 RPMs. Expert cyclists and racers maintain a steady cadence of 90 to 120 RPMs. You can determine your RPMs by timing yourself for a minute while you pedal on level ground. Count the number of times your right knee rises.

Start out by riding in low gears and spinning as fast as you can. You want to feel a little resistance when pedaling but you should not be pushing hard, unless of course you're going uphill. You will not become a good cyclist by pushing hard gears as a novice. Instead, you could be injuring your knees.

The reasons for correct pedaling reflect our overall fitness goals. Rapid, easy pedaling enhances endurance and is non-stressful and pleasurable. It promotes lifetime sports participation.

AVOIDING MINOR HEALTH PROBLEMS

There are some possible cycling health problems you can prevent. I almost despaired and gave up biking because it was becoming a pain in the neck as well as a pain in the bottom. But for me it was because I had the triathlon approaching and was training too hard.

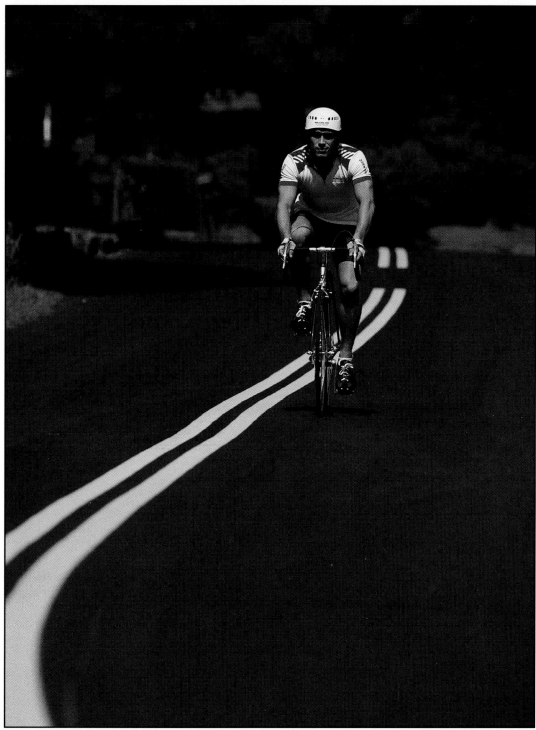

It will probably take you longer to read this chapter about bicycling than it will for you to master riding a bike. A bike is the perfect machine for low-stress exercise and transportation.

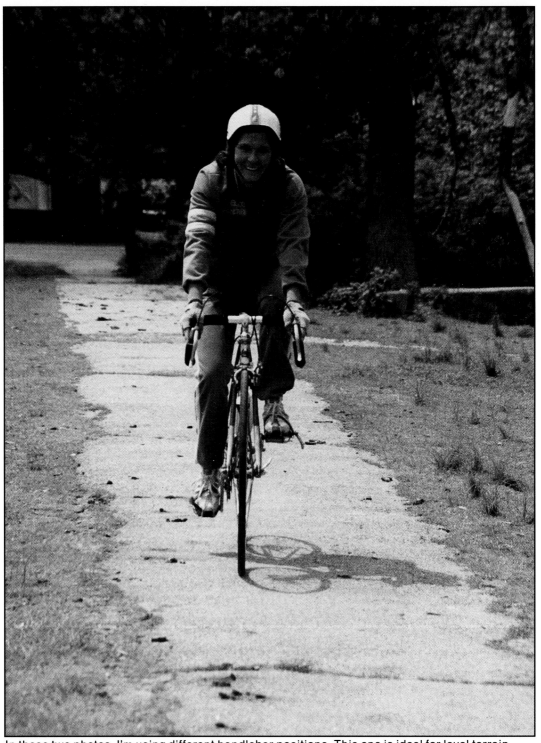

In these two photos, I'm using different handlebar positions. This one is ideal for level terrain.
Photos courtesy of She's A Sport, Inc.

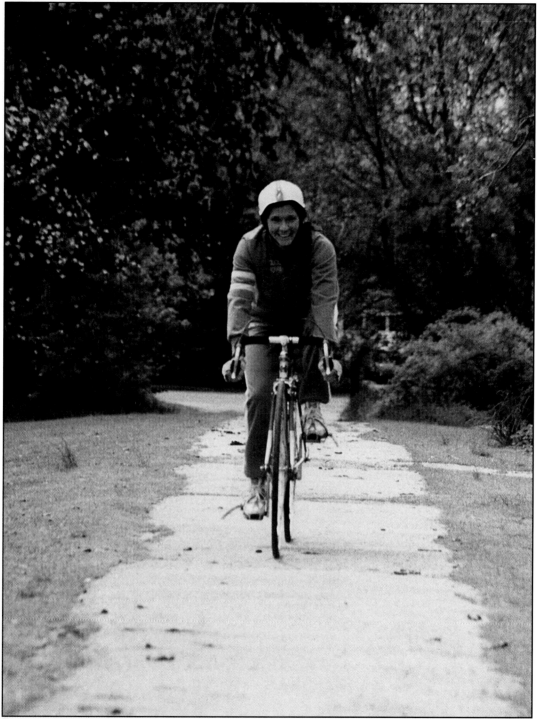

This handlebar position is good when you are riding into the wind. It lowers your upper body a bit, offering a smaller profile to the wind. Some people also use this position during uphill rides when they do "stand-up" pedaling.

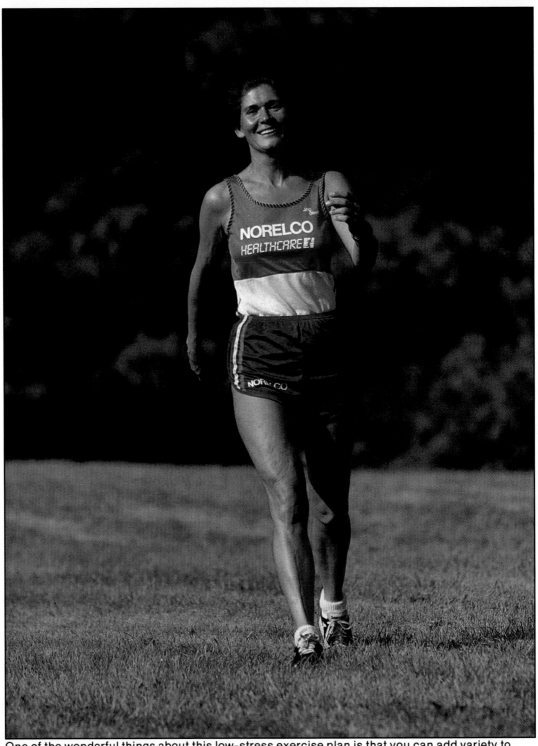

One of the wonderful things about this low-stress exercise plan is that you can add variety to maintain the fun. Chapter 7 describes how you can create your own plan by adding variety.

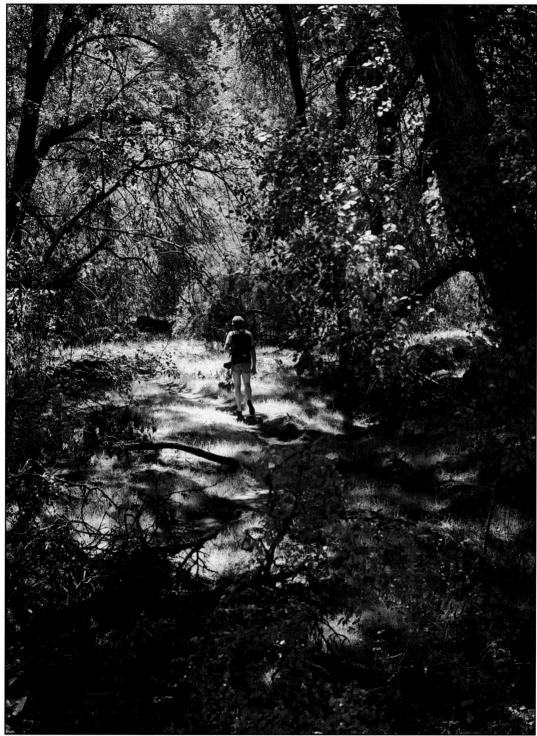

Vary your walks by visiting forests, parks or golf courses. Bicycle country roads, too. Swim in lakes or the ocean. New scenery and sights will motivate you to exercise. Photo by Scott Millard.

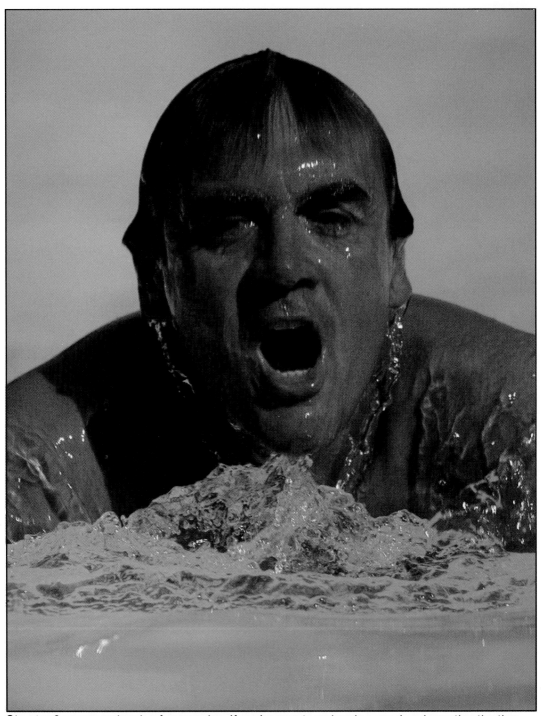

Chapter 6 covers swimming for exercise. If you're new to swimming, read and practice the tips and techniques for getting used to the water and doing the basic crawl stroke. If you need more instruction, or want to learn other strokes such as the breaststroke shown above, join a swimming class at your community pool, "Y" or health club.

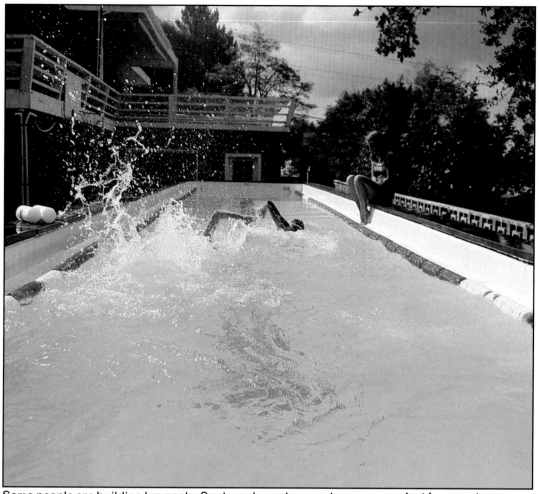

Some people are building lap pools. Such pools are long and narrow—perfect for exercise swimming at home. Photo courtesy of Fastlane Pools, Santa Cruz, CA.

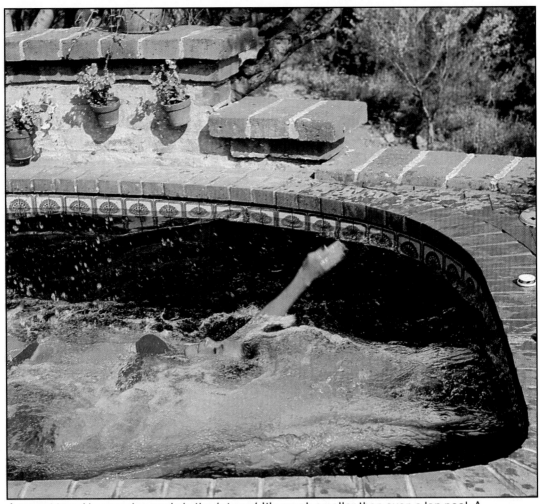

A recent trend in exercise pools is the *jet pool*. It's much smaller than even a lap pool. A high-powered jet stream creates a current that you swim against. Photo courtesy of Patio Pools, Tucson, AZ.

Take It Easy—Your unconditioned muscles will grow stronger. As mentioned in chapter 3, stretching before and after bicycling is very important. Refer to the stretching exercises on page 146.

Upper Body—Avoid or alleviate discomfort in the neck, back and hands by frequently changing hand positions on the handlebars. Also, padded handlebars and gloves are a tremendous help in providing comfort for your hands.

According to research done by Eugene Sloane, "Persons with back pains in the lower lumbar region may also have pains while riding their bikes, but physicians who write on bicycling topics have noted that although no formal studies have been done, the indications are that major back pain is more often relieved rather than aggravated by cycling. Score another one for exercise."

Lower Body—One form of *saddle soreness* starts as chafing caused by friction between the skin and underwear. The other type results from sitting on tissues that are not "toughened" for such use.

These are the handlebar positions used by most bicyclists. As mentioned in the text, changing the position of your hands is a good way to alleviate any discomfort.

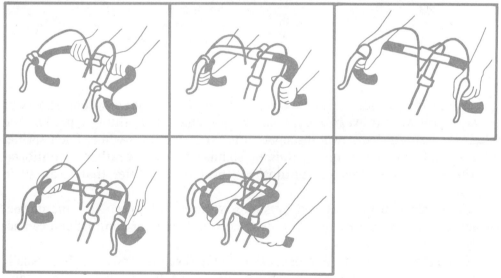

STRETCHES FOR BICYCLING

Exercise #	Name
1	Standing Body Stretch
3	Head Rolls
4	Calf Muscle
5	Achilles Tendon
6	Stork Stretch
8	Side Quad and Leg Stretch
9	Sitting Quad Stretch
10	Hip and Upper Thigh
11	Standing Hamstring Stretch
12	Sitting Hamstring Stretch
13	Forward Bend
14	Groin Stretch
15	Squat
17	Standing Upper Body and Back
21	Upper Spine and Neck
23	Spinal Twist
24	Cat Back
27	Toes and Feet
29	Ankles
30	Calf and Heel
33	Upper Back Hug

Avoid the former by not wearing underwear with good cycling shorts or pants. If you want to wear underwear, wear a small, snug-fitting type. For the latter, be assured that it will disappear after you ride for a while. Each spring, after limited winter rides on my training stand, I have a few rather uncomfortable rides. I refer to those as putting in "butt time." After that I can sit in comfort.

Foot pain is usually caused by shoes without stiff soles. As I mentioned earlier, wearing proper cycling clothes greatly adds to your comfort and can actually prevent problems.

Knee strain is about the most serious injury cycling can cause. It is usually caused by stressing knees too much by excessive riding in high gears. I can't overemphasize the importance of riding in comfortable gears. Try not to go up hills at the beginning of your ride. Give yourself plenty of time in low gears to warm up adequately before riding up hill or in high gears.

Too many exercisers become overzealous in their desire to shape up quickly. Remember, this is a low-stress plan. Take it slowly and easily in the beginning. If you notice pain on the outside or inside of your knee, change the position of your foot slightly so it is straighter on the pedal.

Leg cramps can be caused by pushing high gears and overexertion. If that happens, rest and massage the cramps. Leg and knee pain can also result if your bicycle is not adjusted properly for you.

Weather Precautions—Another warning I must give in regard to safe biking is not to ride in severe weather conditions. If you do, take precautions. In the cold, consider the added wind-chill factor caused by your cycling. Dress warmly in layers.

Riding in the rain is dangerous because of bad visibility, slippery roads, and compromised braking.

As far as heat and wind are concerned, I can give you a first-hand report from my 1983 Ironman experience in Hawaii. The winds were a record high for race day. The winds intensified in the early afternoon as the slower competitors inched their way to the 50-mile turn-around point.

We had a 5-mile hill to climb, fighting an intense headwind all of the way. At one point, it was much too difficult to stay on my bike, so I walked myself and bicycle into the wind. A forceful gust caught another rider head on, picked up him and his bike and threw them backward onto the pavement.

The heat in the lava fields was so intense that I had to drink water every 10 minutes. Just reaching for the water bottle was a harrowing experience. Several times I was blown from one side of the road to the other. And to make matters worse, that year some weirdo scattered tacks on the bike course.

The only reason I did not drop out of the race was because ABC-TV was featuring me, and I knew millions of people would be watching. I was afraid that if I quit, people would think that 40-year-old women aren't capable of such feats.

But that was a unique situation. There is a time to quit and a time to cycle. My advice is to beware of the wind and don't push yourself too hard.

CONCLUSION

Chapter 7 reiterates this a bit more. It discusses ways to bicycle for exercise. In addition, it describes how you can combine biking, walking and swimming for good health.

CHAPTER SIX

Swimming

The same week I had my bicycle accident I had another frightening experience—this one involved swimming. I had waded out to a raft 100 feet off shore at a local beach to sun myself. As I enjoyed the sun, the tide came in. I was forced to swim—not wade—back to shore. I swam for the first 15 feet then panicked. I thrashed and yelled until the lifeguard pulled me to shore.

EARLY WATER DAYS

How could this be? I grew up around the water and loved it. As a child I imitated my older brother. He swam, so I learned how to swim. He water skied, so I took up the sport. When he earned his Red Cross Life Saving Certicate, I went after the Junior Certificate.

After I married, I moved away from the water. My idea of going to the beach and swimming consisted of lying in the sun and wading into the water.

The only explanation I had for my new fear of the water was that I was getting older. While I could accept the gray hair and wrinkles that came with maturity, I found it hard to accept the loss of courage my birthdays seemed to bring.

I signed up for beginning swimming at the YMCA and felt like crying when I couldn't make it across the pool. Yet two years later I was on the beach in Hawaii preparing for my 2-1/2-mile swim in the Ironman competition.

This chapter is filled with tips on how you can learn, or re-learn, to swim to fitness. Perhaps conquering the challenge and becoming a swimmer will enable you to overcome a crisis in your life.

Maybe I'll swim the English Channel when I'm 80! I don't anticipate any more aging problems for at least 30 years.

SWIMMING'S THERAPEUTIC EFFECTS

Swimming is one of the most popular sports in America. It allows you to exercise major skeletal muscles without risking injury. It is considered the best exercise to tone shoulders, arms, waistline, hips and legs—all at the same time. Muscles become elongated and strengthened, increasing your range of motion and flexibility.

In addition, swimming permits a relatively *higher cardiac output* because your body is horizontal and supported by water. Because the heart doesn't have to pump against gravity, it pumps between 10% and 20% more with each contraction. As a result, you can exercise longer and harder than you could on land.

Swimming helps alleviate problems associated with varicose veins. The veins are massaged and tightened with every movement in the water. Swelling and enlargement decreases because the pressure is much less in the veins when you swim.

Who Benefits Most—Doctors often recommend swimming for people recovering from illness because of the way it builds physical and mental stamina. Swimming is especially recommended for *cardiac patients* because it is less strenuous and more soothing than many other exercises.

Chiropractors, orthopedists and osteopathic physicians recommend swimming for patients suffering from *back ailments* because water bears most of the body weight. Many people crippled with *arthritis* have also improved through exercising in the water. It's a great way to exercise without straining.

Overweight people also find swimming more comfortable than any other form of exercise. The support of the water helps, but overweight people are also more buoyant than thin people. In a lifesaving course I took several years ago there was an overweight woman and eight lanky teenage boys. It was much easier to practice lifesaving carries or tows on the woman than the boys. She floated; they sank. That woman, by the way, is no longer overweight after several years of lap swimming.

Women have excelled in *endurance* swimming probably because of their body composition. Distribution of body fat in women is such that legs float high in the water, making them more "streamlined." Men's leaner legs tend to swing down and float lower in the water, increasing body drag and reducing swimming efficiency.

Cooling Effect—A benefit of exercising in the water is the cooling effect of water. Exercise generates heat, but water cools body temperature immediately and prevents serious overheating. Overweight people who find working out painful and uncomfortable will find relief through swimming.

Caloric Effect—Swimming will increase your metabolism and is a good way to burn off calories. Depending on your speed, time, stroke and weight, you can burn between 300 and 700 calories an hour. A reasonable estimate for even a slow swimmer would be approximately eight calories burned per minute. Additionally, many swimmers report a decrease in appetite after vigorous swims.

Swimmer's "High"—Swimming has definite therapeutic effects on the mind. The water can create a state of *altered sensory perception,* muffling sounds and making movement appear in slow motion. Thinking is directed inward, especially when you swim in a pool where the surroundings are safe, familiar and relatively constant. The combined effects of the water and the regular rhythmical action create a restfulness unlike other exercises. This relaxation also carries into post-swim activities.

The Sensual Exercise—Swimming can have another positive effect on you—it can improve your sex life. Researchers find that swimming affects the body's hormonal balance and can temporarily produce a greater sexual appreciation. Match that with the endurance, energy, graceful movements and improved self-esteem you get from swimming, and you will understand why I consider it the most sensual of exercises.

It made my life much more pleasurable, and it can do the same for you. You don't need much to get started, so let's swim!

EQUIPMENT

The only essential equipment is a suit, cap and goggles. I mentioned in the cycling section the advantages of proper clothing and equipment, and the same reasoning applies here.

Goggles—Goggles should be worn by anyone who swims in chlorine or saltwater pools. Although opthalmologists say that chlorine will cause no irreversible damage to the eye, most people feel a burning sensation after exposure. Also, eyes can become bloodshot from pool chemicals or saltwater. Goggles prevent this irritation.

Goggles should fit snugly, but if they are too tight they can cause headaches. You can typically adjust the centerpiece over the nose and the rubber headband for comfort.

Goggles are available in a variety of lens colors, including clear. Yellow and rose-colored lenses tend to make indoor light seem brighter. If you will be swimming in bright sunlight, the gray, blue or green tints will help shield your eyes best. If you have bad eyesight, *prescription* goggles are also available.

Fogging can be annoying. If that's a problem for you, try anti-fog goggles. De-fogging preparations are available, but be sure to apply the stuff sparingly and rinse the goggles well before wearing them. The chemical can get into your eyes and cause burning.

I had to drop out of a triathlon because the de-fog solution in my goggles irritated my eyes and gave me vision problems during the bike segment. Now to prevent fogging I moisten my goggles with saliva, a trick swimmers and divers have been using for years. It will take a little time to become accustomed to your goggles, but it is well worth it. You wear them *over* your swim cap.

Swim Caps—A swim cap will not keep your hair dry, but it will protect your hair from the chemicals. Ladies, resist the temptation to wear the swim cap you purchased 15 years ago, especially if it is bulky, bouffant or has a chin strap. Old-style caps will date you, and the chin strap could cause chafing. Those old caps are not very streamlined. A new, sleek rubber or lycra cap costs only a few dollars.

Swim Suits—The best suits for swimming are made of nylon or Lycra. I recommend a one-piece tank or maillot-type suit for women. Racing suits have straps placed strategically to provide the greatest freedom of movement. Don't use suits decorated with ruffles, buckles and bows because they create drag in the water and make swimming harder.

When buying a suit, be alert for seams that could irritate your skin. I learned that the hard way. At the end of a mile swim I found that a rough seam of my suit had worn through my skin.

Kickboards—A kickboard is a good piece of *training* equipment. It's a U-shaped rectangular slab made of compressed plastic or foam. You can find a good one for about $7.

With it you can keep your face out of the water while you practice or strengthen your kick. You hold the board out in front of you, the rounded part forward. Your feet should just barely churn the surface of the water when you kick.

Duffle Bag—Keep a duffle bag with your swim equipment packed and in view, as a reminder to swim frequently. In it have your suit, goggles, cap, shampoo, conditioning rinse, soap, moisturizing lotion and two towels.

THE TIME AND PLACE TO SWIM

Swimming is not just a hot-weather sport any more, now that there are so many indoor pools. YMCA and YWCA pools are great places to swim. They usually have large pools with designated lap swims and are often open from early morning until late evening. There is always a lifeguard on duty. Also, swim classes at the "Y" are usually reasonably priced.

Check your area for health clubs, hotels, parks and recreation department, high schools, colleges and municipal sports centers for pool availability. You may even have a friend or neighbor who has a pool and would welcome a swimming companion. There are 1.5 million indoor and outdoor swimming pools in the country, plus 2 million above-ground portable pools. In addition, it is estimated that 80,000 new pools are built every year.

Safety Advice—In warm weather it's great to swim outdoors, but select a site designed for swimming. Otherwise the safe, injury-free sport of swimming can be very dangerous. I suggest that you *never swim alone!* It's always best to swim where there is a lifeguard or other swimmers around. Unsupervised swimming in rivers, ponds, quarries, lakes and ocean beaches can expose you to unpredictable and dangerous hazards.

Of course, the safest, most relaxed area to learn to swim is in a pool with shallow water, especially if you have *any* fear of the water.

Start the Day Swimming—An early morning swim before work is a great way to start the day. Wear a sweatsuit over your swimsuit and take your work clothes with you. I guarantee that an invigorating swim will be more effective than coffee to perk you up.

A lot of people swim laps at lunchtime, which gives them added energy for the afternoon. A swim after work is a marvelous way to wash away the tensions of a difficult day. I'm lucky to have a flexible schedule. I like to swim late mornings or early afternoons when the pool is almost deserted. Or I'll swim in the evening, rather than sit in front of the TV and snack.

If you have young children, you could exchange babysitting time with another mother to get a break to go swimming. The pool or "Y" may have babysitting, or there may be fitness programs for kids that coincide with your swims. If the kids are old enough, take them with you. Swim between your car pooling: Drop the kids at their practice, enjoy your swim, then pick them up.

Even if you can fit in swimming only once a week, make the effort to find the time and place. I think you'll learn to love the sport. Then you may find yourself scheduling other activities around your swim!

SWIMMING SAFELY

You should stretch before and after your swim. The accompanying table shows which stretches from chapter 3 I recommend you do.

I can't overemphasize that you should never swim alone. And swim only with a person who could help you if necessary. When training for the Ironman, I had to do long swims in the ocean. At my local beach I would swim parallel to the shore in shallow water.

When practicing the swim course in Hawaii, I would do it with other athletes. But I always had my inner tube tied to my ankle. It created some drag

STRETCHES FOR SWIMMING

Exercise #	Name
1	Standing Body Stretch
8	Side Quad and Leg Stretch
14	Groin Stretch
15	Squat
16	Iliopsoas Lunge
17	Standing Upper Body and Back
18	Upper Body
19	Upper Body With Towel
20	Shoulder Stretch
21	Upper Spine and Neck
25	Kneeling Spine Stretch
29	Ankles
33	Upper Back Hug
34	Overall Body Stretch

but gave me a lot of security. In the event of an emergency I did not want to have to depend on another tired swimmer.

Know your limitations and don't overestimate your ability.

Cramps—If you're overheated, don't jump into cool water. That could cause cramps, a concern for many swimmers. Although studies have dispelled the myth about staying out of the water after a meal, it is still recommended not to eat heavily before a strenuous swim.

Muscle cramps usually occur in the legs, feet or hands. The cramp is the effect of sudden muscle tightening. If you feel a cramp coming on, *change your movement.* Stop and relax.

If you develop a cramp, do not pound the muscle. Instead, *stretch and knead* the area with your thumbs. Alternate between direct pressure and relaxation until the cramp goes away. Don't panic. Try to relax until it passes.

Coughing—Water in the nose or unexpectedly swallowed can cause coughing. Stop, stay calm and force a few strong coughs to clear things up.

Short Breath—Shortness of breath is usually an indication that the body's capacity is being overtaxed. In this case, slow down. Try to relax and breathe *evenly.* Breathing that is too shallow does not exchange oxygen and carbon dioxide efficiently. Conversely, respiratory muscles will tire from breathing that is too deep. If you become very anxious and panicky, you may find yourself gasping for air. The key is to *relax.*

Hypothermia—Do not stay long in chilly water. If you begin shivering, or if toes or fingers feel numb or blue, you may be approaching *hypothermia.* It's a dangerous condition marked by rapidly falling body temperature. *Get out of the water immediately and warm up.*

OVERCOMING FEARS AND ANXIETIES

Many people have a fear of the water. No one is born with it. Rather, it usually results from a traumatic childhood experience. Often parents who are afraid of the water instill this fear in their children. Sometimes, fears develop as we grow older, as mine did, because of a general lack of confidence.

Fearful non-swimmers can be gripped by a very specific and intense terror. They are afraid of being helpless in a large body of water.

No matter how intense your fear of water, the best way to overcome it is to learn to swim. You should learn in a very relaxed, secure setting where the water is shallow and a friend or lifeguard is nearby. Put no time restrictions on yourself. You don't need the pressure of a deadline to overcome a fear.

You should also try to determine what your specific fears are, rather than the obvious fear of drowning. You may have a specific fear of choking, not being able to see, getting water in your nose or not being able to breathe. The fear may be of losing your balance, falling, or not having something solid to hold onto in the water. You may have a fear of a few or all of these things.

Until you overcome them, you will have a serious problem learning to swim in the conventional manner.

I'll outline some specialized instructions aimed at overcoming your fears. You can practice some of these in your bathtub, sink, a basin or on dry land. You should try to locate a lake, shallow water at a beach, or an outdoor pool. The bottom should slope very gradually and should be smooth enough to sit on. Practice there in the summertime to overcome your fear of large bodies of water. Rivers can be dangerous because of currents and drop-offs. The ocean will be too rough.

Don't use a life jacket or flotation aid because you will develop a dependency on them. Make sure there are lifeguards, attentive swimmers, or friends nearby.

Water Familiarity—Getting into the water may be a big obstacle if you are terrified of it. As mentioned before, find a safe, supervised lake or pool where there is plenty of shallow water. Wade into the water up to your knees and sit down. Relax and enjoy yourself.

The idea is to become *comfortable* in the water. Feel the bottom; lean forward and backward. The water should not be so deep at this point that it reaches your armpits. It may take weeks or months to become familiar with and at ease in a large body of water.

If you have been afraid of the water for a long time, your fear will not go away in one day. The main thing is to work on overcoming it now, so you can enjoy it for the rest of your life. If I did it, you can too.

Moving Around—The next step is to crawl around in the water on your hands and knees. Then stretch legs out in back of you and support your weight with your arms about a foot apart. Your head and top of shoulders should be out of the water. Work on this exercise as long as it takes to become comfortable and secure in this position.

Then, instead of dragging your legs behind you, start moving them slowly up and down in a kick. Pretend you're swimming, but stay where it is shallow enough to walk on your hands with your head out of the water. Take a lot of time in this position looking out into the deeper water, convincing yourself there is nothing to fear.

Some experts advocate that you learn the whole swimming process in knee-deep water. While this is a good idea, inflatable kiddie pools and the bathtub will not resolve your fear of larger bodies of deep water. Learn to swim and build your confidence in the shallow area of the water. When you achieve that, your confidence will soar. I did and still do a lot of my long-distance swims in very shallow water parallel to the shore.

Those of you without an intense fear of water can get in the pool in chest-deep water. Hold on to the side of the pool and practice bobbing and breathing, as shown in the following photos.

BREATHING

Correct, relaxed breathing while swimming is challenging for most people. I've heard many people say, "I can swim, but for the life of me I can't get the breathing right." Consequentially, they swim in short, tiring spurts and don't enjoy the sport. If you can just master deep, relaxed breathing with the rotation of your head in and out of the water, your swimming will *immediately* improve 50%.

The best techniques I've found for breathing practice can be done at home. These are adapted from *Swimming for Total Fitness* by Jane Katz. You will become relaxed as you combine breathing with swimming. And after the practice session at home, you will be less tense. I urge you to try them.

Step One—Sit up straight. Inhale, fully expanding your lungs, then exhale. Remember how it feels to have your lungs really full because they should feel this way every time you take a breath in the water.

Now, hold your nostrils shut, pucker your lips and inhale strongly through your mouth as if you were drinking through a straw. Then, with lips still puckered, strongly *exhale* through your mouth as if you were cooling off some hot soup. Blow into your hand so you can feel the air. Concentrate on making your inhalation and exhalation cycles strong and rhythmic. Try to maintain a

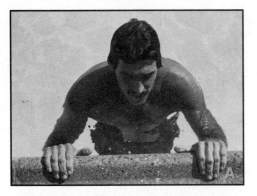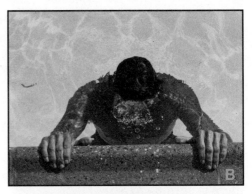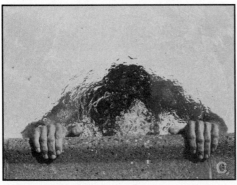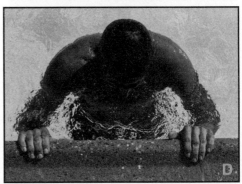

Take a breath (A). Bend your knees and lower your entire body in the water (B). Be sure to submerge your head. Keep your eyes open and exhale through your mouth and nose, making a constant stream of air bubbles (C). Raise your head back above the surface, keeping your hands on the side of the pool (D). Avoid the tendency to wipe the water from your face. Take a deep breath when your head is above the water and exhale deeply underwater. Practice this about eight times.

steady stream of air for 10 seconds. Repeat this eight times, taking very deep breaths.

Step Two—Close your mouth and inhale deeply through your nose. Then exhale, expelling the air strongly. Repeat eight times.

Step Three—Practice inhaling deeply through both your nose *and* mouth, and exhaling forcefully. Repeat eight times.

Be aware of using your nose in these breathing exercises. In the water people naturally tend to exhale through the mouth, but you should learn to exhale correctly out of both your nose and mouth at the same time. This prevents water from getting in breathing passages. Be sure not to swim with your mouth closed. Nasal passages are too small to bear the intense pressure of underwater exhalation.

The point to remember about breathing in swimming is to inhale very deeply through both your mouth and nose when your face is out of the water.

When your head is underwater, blow out hard through nose and mouth to create a protective air flow.

Add Some Water—Now, I'll explain a way to practice proper breathing in water at home. This way you'll have already developed good breathing habits before you swim.

Fill a large container with water. The sink, bathtub, a big bowl or basin will do. Leaning forward, barely touch your chin to the surface of the water. Inhale using both your nose and mouth. Take a very deep breath. Then exhale through both your nose and mouth, watching the water for ripples to form on the surface. If the water stays calm, you need to exhale harder. The water should form ripples each time you exhale. Repeat this eight times.

Practice inhaling through your nose and mouth together. Put your face in the water and exhale strongly through both your nose and mouth. Bubbles should form, indicating proper air flow. You'll be able to see, hear and feel the bubbles.

When all the air is exhaled, lift your nose and mouth out of the water and inhale deeply. Repeat eight times without stopping.

Now, put your whole face in the water and exhale. On the inhalation phase, turn to the right as if lying on a pillow, so your nose and mouth are out of the water. Take a large breath, put your face back into the water and exhale as strongly as you can. Alternate by taking your next breath on the left side. Continue this alternating breathing as long as you can.

Aim for *total relaxation* while doing this exercise. When you exhale, think of releasing all your tensions. Let your muscles relax and go limp. By practicing this exercise at home, breathing in the water will soon be second nature.

KICKING

Sit on the side of the pool with your feet in the water and practice the flutter kick. You can also practice this at home by sitting on the edge of a couch or a chair with your legs straight out in front of you.

Points to remember when kicking are to keep your toes pointed downward, ankles relaxed and knees straight. Be sure you kick with your whole leg, using power from the hip and thigh. Alternate your legs up and down with a space of about 10 inches between your feet. Practice this at a moderate pace about 20 times.

Practice in the Water—Now, practice the kick while in the water and holding on to the side of the pool. One hand should hold on to the edge of the pool. The other hand is underwater, pressing against the wall with your fingers pointed down. Keep your arms straight for leverage by pushing with the lower arm and pulling with the upper one. Your feet should be close together near the water surface.

Move your legs up and down as you did on dry land, keeping your legs straight but not stiff. Be sure you kick from the hip and thighs. Your feet should not be coming out of the water, creating a large splash. If they are, you are overkicking. You want to achieve a constant churning action. Practice this for a few minutes, then practice your breathing, too, as you kick.

GLIDE AND KICK

Hold on to a kickboard with your arms straight out in front of you. Stand at the side of the pool on one foot. Use the other foot to push yourself away from the wall. Inhale, put your head face down in the water and exhale while you kick. Turn your face to the side and inhale, remembering the breathing techniques you practiced at home.

Keep relaxed and build confidence as you practice kicking and breathing. Go back and forth in the pool, stretching your arms and legs so your body is streamlined.

If you not making much progress, it could be because you are bending your knees too much or because your toes are not pointed.

CRAWL STROKE

The most common swim stroke is the *Australian crawl,* sometimes called just the *crawl.* You can practice this stroke while using your kickboard, concentrating on one arm, then the other. The stroke consists of the arm *pull and recovery.*

Pull Technique—Start the stroke by extending your arm in front of you so it enters the water in line with the top of your shoulder. Your thumb enters the water first with your hand at a 45° angle. Avoid placing your hand flat against the surface of the water because that will cause air bubbles and lower the efficiency of the arm pull.

As soon as the hand is in the water, turn it so the palm is facing the bottom of the pool. Pull your arm under your body, bending your elbow until it forms a 90° angle under your shoulder.

Your hand should trace a zig-zag pattern as you pull it down and back under your body. Position your hand so you feel a constant pressure on your palms as your hand pulls against the water. This creates the force that propels you through the water.

It is very important to keep your elbow high in the first half of the pull. Do this by bending the elbow and keeping it almost stationary as you press your hand downward. If you let your elbow drop, you will use up energy without making much progress.

Continue to pull your hand to a midline point of your body and then pass

158

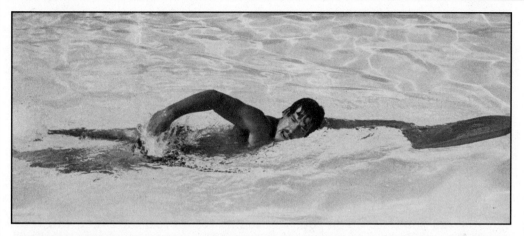

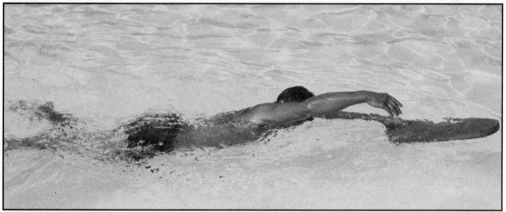

This is the basic arm motion of the crawl stroke. You can practice it with a kickboard until you master the stroke.

the bottom of your swim suit. You will finish the pull with your elbow almost straight and the palm of your hand back behind your hips.

Arm Recovery—The recovery phase is the movement of the hand from behind your hips until it enters the water again outstretched in front of your shoulders.

Keep your elbow as high as you can as you bring your arm forward. Bend the elbow slightly as your arm comes out of the water. When your arm swings forward, elbow bend increases. Keep the elbow high as your hand clears the water. Keep your hand close to your body, no more than a few inches out of the water, as you bring it forward. Avoid swinging the arm too wide with a straight elbow. That will make your hips wiggle.

Your elbow begins to extend as your arm reaches forward. Your elbow is is almost fully extended as your hand re-enters the water for the "catch" or start of the next arm pull. Try to keep the elbow higher than the hand during the arm recovery.

Repeat these arm movements, concentrating on the proper placement with the support of the kickboard. Then, bend over in waist-high water and practice coordinating the right and left arm. When you have mastered that, you can simultaneously practice correct breathing in that position.

Breathing for the Crawl Stroke—I strongly recommend *alternate breathing* because it helps you swim a straighter course. It enables you to see on both sides as you swim.

The best way to coordinate alternate breathing with your arm strokes is to take a breath on your *right side* when your left arm is extended. Count two arm strokes as your head is down exhaling. On the third stroke as your right arm extends, roll your face up on your *left,* and inhale. Repeat the count with your head coming up on the third count on the opposite side.

When breathing, do not lift your head high and straight out of the water. That will lower your legs and slow down your forward movement. Turn your head *to the side* as if it were on a swivel and take the breath when your body is at its maximum roll to the side.

The proper timing of head movement in relation to the arm stroke occurs when the hand on the breathing side is beginning its recovery.

Keep in mind that air is exhaled almost continuously while your face is underwater. Don't hold your breath when swimming. Keep your breathing rhythmical and relaxed. The air should slowly trickle out of your nose and mouth at the first part of the exhalation. As you tilt your head toward the surface, blow out explosively. This action gets rid of any air left in your lungs and also forces water away from your mouth so you can inhale without sucking in water.

The main reason swimmers become fatigued is an inadequate supply of oxygen. When you master the ability to stay relaxed while breathing fully and deeply, swimming will become simple, and you won't tire.

I practiced my breathing in the security of my bathtub and within a short period of time my swimming distances increased many, many times.

Head Position—Your aim is to keep your body as streamlined as possible in the water. Your head should not be too high or too low. The water should break at about the middle of your forehead, and your elbows should not be out of the water. While swimming, look forward and diagonally down at about a 45° angle.

Don't be overwhelmed and think it's too complicated to coordinate the arm movement, breathing and kick. Practice them separately, concentrating on each aspect.

OTHER STROKES

Your swimming workouts will be more fun if you incorporate a variety of strokes. Try to spend a lot of your time and energy mastering the crawl stroke. It is the best stroke for achieving relaxation and the "swimmer's high." But you can also use the sidestroke, backstroke or breaststroke. However, it's probably easier to learn these—including the crawl—by taking an introductory swimming class at your local "Y" or community pool.

When you start swimming, relax as much as possible. Don't worry about form. If you have practiced each movement separately, unconcious patterns will have formed. Let your body take over. Banish negative thoughts of all kinds. Swim and relax. Swim and enjoy.

Chapter 7 stresses this theme too. It discusses ways to swim for exercise. In addition, it describes how you can combine swimming, walking and biking for good health.

Creating Your Low-Stress-Fitness Plan

The previous three chapters discussed specific types of exercise, but didn't give you a clear way to train. That's the job of this chapter. It outlines workouts for walking, cycling and swimming at beginner and intermediate levels. You will also find a plan showing how you can combine all of the exercises in one week's plan. From that you can customize a low-stress fitness plan of your own.

GENERAL ADVICE

Go at your own pace without feeling that you have to race constantly. Instead, try to push yourself a little farther and a little faster at the midpoint of each workout. This gives a beneficial training effect.

My theory is that if you acquire a love of the sport, you will want to do it the rest of your life. I would rather you take longer to reach the desired heart rate and distance—enjoying the sport as you go—than to have you build to your fitness level quickly and lose interest.

Listen to your body. When you're feeling listless, don't push. Go slowly, keeping your body relaxed and in motion. On the days you feel vigorous, push yourself a bit and work on increasing speed and endurance. You will probably feel tired a day or so after a hard workout. That's normal, so be sure to give yourself some easy days.

Do try to make some form of exercise a daily habit, even if all you do is stretch.

MEASURING PROGRESS

Keep records, such as on a weekly engagement calendar, to chart regular progress. This gives you a great sense of accomplishment. You can look back and marvel at your advancement over a period of time.

For some people, recording the workout provides an incentive and sharpens discipline. In the last six years of training, I have found a consensus: Everyone I have talked to stresses record-keeping.

My Own Record—I must admit that this is one area where I don't practice what I preach. I *have* bought a lot of elaborate exercise log and record books, but I rarely write in them—something I sometimes regret.

During serious training, I felt guilty because I didn't keep track of my distances. When an interviewer would ask, "How many miles do you put in?," I would fumble for an answer.

A running friend was appalled that after four years of racing I didn't know my best 10K time. "That's unheard of in the running world!" he said.

Undocumented Relaxation—Occasionally I would win a race and set a personal record, but to me the true success was having a fun, relaxed time. I started to notice that my fastest race times resulted when I simply went out to have fun.

Over the years I have developed what I call a "relaxed push" kind of training. This is the 25% of my exercise time when I push my body a little farther and a little faster. During this time I focus completely on relaxed breathing and allow only positive, encouraging thoughts. This form of non-stress training, without detailed records, has worked for me.

Conversely, there have been moments of great regret at not having better records of my mileage. One of those times was on a New Year's Day. I was talking with my friend Ted Treu about our accomplishments of the past year and goals for the new year. He told me that in six months of training for the Ironman he documented 114 swim miles, 2,589 bike miles, and 541 running miles.

Ted is a 47-year-old devoted father and busy executive. I was amazed and impressed, but also a little envious. "Darn!" I thought. "Why didn't I record *my* miles?"

What's Best for You—Perhaps it is a matter of personal taste. If you are so inclined, ignore keeping records. If you regard them as a form of stress-inducing regimentation, don't use them. But they can be helpful as guidelines. They can document your growing feeling of accomplishment. And, during low times, they provide encouragement. Whatever your choice, be sure to make exercise a regular part of your life.

MORE ON STRETCHING

Throughout this book I've stressed the importance of stretching—both before and after exercise—as a sport unto its own. You need to make it a habit, to find the appropriate triggers or reminders to motivate you to stretch. Try one of my suggestions or be creative and determine what stimulates you.

- Stretch while watching TV or listening to the radio.
- Have a special exercise outfit you change into to get things moving.
- Try music. I find music stimulating. When faced with dreary household chores, I would make a point of playing my favorite music. I was able to disassociate myself from the task and enjoy myself. For my stretching sessions, I recorded a tape of my favorite music, fitting the tempo of the songs to the exercises.

MORE ON WALKING

Remember Betty Dolen, the "Happy Hoofer" I mentioned in chapter 4? She progressed from walking around her yard to walking the Appalachian Trail, 2,100 miles between Springer Mountain, Georgia, and Mount Katahdin, Maine.

Ten years ago she came to a point where she felt the job of raising kids and taking care of the house would never end. She claims that walking was her salvation because it gave her something to look forward to. "I'm the kind of person," said Betty, "who would have felt very frivolous going out to lunch or playing bridge every day. But walking seemed healthy and productive."

Betty had advanced to walking around the block when a neighbor told her about the Appalachian Mountain Club. She sent away for information and found that she could join groups who walked on the Appalachian Trail.

Day Trips—Heartened to know that she could join other walking enthusiasts and venture out of town, Betty began to have a new look on life. On day trips, she was able to complete all the Connecticut trails. Then she set out to walk the bordering states of New York and Massachusetts.

During one of these walks the "Happy Hoofer" met a woman whose goal was to walk the complete Appalachian Trail. The challenge was contagious.

In the next 10 years, Betty and her walking buddies enjoyed hiking and backpacking on overnights, weekends and week-long treks.

A Healthy Outlook—She inspired countless other people to take up walking as a form of exercise and a source of pleasure. Betty knows she looks good, is healthy, and claims that walking has definitely helped her mental outlook. She now has another important objective in life in addition to taking care of her family.

"Now everyone respects my walking time," she says. "Come hell or high water, I'm going to get in my walk each day. It gets me out of the house with a purposeful objective."

Her husband is an avid runner and very involved in his running club. Betty and some of the other non-running spouses or injured runners have started walking the courses their partners were racing. Her current challenge is to walk the marathon courses her husband completes. She figures it will take her six and one-half hours to walk a marathon.

In fact, that's about how long it took me to do the marathon in the 1983 Ironman. It hurt too much to run, so I walked most of it.

Betty Dolen started walking around her yard and ended up walking the Appalachian Trail. What may seem at the start as a simple, tedious task can turn into an exciting and rewarding challenge.

LOW-STRESS WALKING PLAN

Your height and leg length are factors to consider when calculating how fast you can walk. In walking, one foot stays on the ground while the other extends out. The length of your legs determines how far you can reach with that other leg. A 15-minute mile could require a fast pace for a short person with short legs. A tall person may find a 17-minute mile too slow.

Because of this, you will want to adjust the accompanying workout tables to suit your frame as well as your age and fitness. The important thing to remember is to strive to increase distance and speed.

Pace—The number of weeks or months required will be determined by your temperament. As long as you try to acquire the habit of daily exercise, you are on the path to improvement. Speed and aggressiveness are not measures of success. Persistence and dedication are.

WALKING WORKOUT
(Beginner Level)

Week	Miles	Time (min.)
1	1	comfortable pace
2	1	17
3	1	15
4	1-1/2	23
5	2	33
6	2-1/2	38
7	2-3/4	45
8	3	50
9	3	47
10	3-1/4	52
11	3-1/2	55
12	3-1/2	52

WALKING WORKOUT
(Intermediate Level)

Week	Miles	Time (min.)
1	3-3/4	56
2	4	62
3	4	60
4	4-1/4	64
5	4-1/2	70
6	4-1/2	68
7	4-3/4	73
8	4-3/4	72
9	5	75
10	5-1/4	80
11	5-1/2	83
12	6	90

My reason for making the accompanying plan easy is so you won't feel compelled to push too hard, too soon and consequently burn out. There will come a point in your progress where you may want to challenge yourself. The plan can address that level of performance.

Physically and mentally you will be able to reach that new plateau without feeling stressed. You will have good inner feelings of accomplishment and at that point you can make "great strides."

LOW-STRESS BICYCLING PLAN

I think my experiences of the past few years proves that our lives can change and improve drastically. Things that now might seem a drudgery can become easy and enjoyable as your fitness level improves. I have met hundreds of middle-aged and older people who now enjoy sports they once considered impossible. Many agree that bicycling offers the widest variety for fun and adventure.

There are bicycle clubs in almost every city. Cyclists are of all ages, abilities and types. I've developed tremendous friendships with people I've met through sport clubs. There is usually a cross-section of income and educational levels, yet there seems to be an equality among members. They love their sport and are eager to share their experiences and expertise with others.

Choose Your Group—Inquire at bicycle shops about the types of bicycle clubs in your area. Some may cater to recreational fun rides, touring or racing. Be sure you check out their goals and the types of rides scheduled. If you are interested in a 10-mile leisurely ride that includes a picnic, you don't want to join a racing club interested in riding 40 miles in two hours.

Rewards of Touring—Through the bike clubs you may meet people who spend their vacations touring on bicycles. Travel agents and bicycling magazines have brochures on organized bicycle tours in different areas of this country and abroad. Some tours feature a "sag wagon"—an accompanying vehicle that carries luggage and an occasional tired biker. Some tour groups camp; others stay in hotels or inns.

You can select the area, type of terrain, price range—whatever suits your tastes. Work on improving your bicycle skills in a leisurely and enjoyable fashion. In a few years you may have the time of your life on a bicycle vacation.

The tourers I know unanimously enjoy bicycle touring, claiming it's a great way to sightsee. They say food tastes better after a few hours of cycling, and they rest better at night. The best reward is that at the end their vacation they show a weight loss and a resurge of vitality.

Commuting—If you're the practical type and the circumstances are right, consider adopting cycling as a means of transportation. Commuting by bike can keep you healthy while saving money and adding less pollutants to the environment.

The U.S. Department of Transportation estimates that there are 2-1/2 million bike commuters. The city of Washington, D.C., has approximately 70,000 people commuting regularly by bike. In Denver, 25,000 commuters cycle to work on extensive paths and bike routes set up by city traffic and transportation planners. Thief-proof bicycle racks are also provided by the city.

One expert points to a study on bicycle commuting in Chicago. The study showed the average commute by car to be 6.9 miles at 22 miles per hour—a trip of 19 minutes. The same trip on a bicycle at 12 miles per hour took 34 minutes. But the time difference narrows when you consider that the car has to be warmed up, can be caught in traffic jams and must be parked.

Economic Advantages—The cost of upkeep on a bicycle is less than one penny a mile. Some car-rental agencies estimate the cost of operating an auto to be 50 cents per mile! Gas prices, higher insurance payments, expensive maintenance and repairs, and parking fees or fines may compel you to think about bicycle commuting.

It is estimated that for every million bicycle commuters, 3.2 million barrels of oil per year are saved. These cyclists not only protect their own lungs and health, but also help the nation by conserving energy resources and not polluting the air.

You may be thinking, "I'll be polluting my office if I bike to work because I'll stink." If you're lucky enough to work at a company with shower and locker

FROM BED TO BIKE:
THE STORY OF JOHN MARINO

To clear up the misconception that biking causes back problems, I'm going to tell you of one of the country's top cyclists, John Marino.

INJURY AND DECLINE

In his early 20s John hurt himself while lifting weights. He suffered a severe compression fracture of his lower lumbar vertebrae. His doctors told him he had a permanent disability and would be severely restricted for the rest of his life. His budding baseball career with the Los Angeles Dodgers ended, and for the next five years his physical and mental state declined. He gave up exercise and consoled himself with food. He gained weight and became lethargic.

THE LONG ROAD BACK

John finally met a doctor who urged him to stop looking for miracle cures and start taking care of himself. The doctor convinced John that the human body has tremendous regenerative powers. The prescription for getting John's body back to health started with diet—low fat, no sugar, no alcohol, no refined food products, no red meat and no tobacco.

Though he was skeptical at first, he followed the recommendations to the letter, and his body began to respond. For the first time in years he allowed himself to think about being active in sports again.

THE EXERCISE PLAN

John needed a gentle exercise that wouldn't stress his back. When a friend suggested bicycling, John knew that he found what he needed. He started riding only one to two miles a day.

The more he rode, the better he felt. And, the better he felt, the more he wanted to ride. Soon he was riding 10 to 20 miles at a time. His back eventually relaxed, and the painful muscle spasms that once kept him a slave to his injuries began to subside. He has since become one of America's most inspiring cyclists.

WARNING

Remember that John was under a doctor's care and advice. Also, his progress didn't happen overnight. You shouldn't let physical weaknesses or problems become excuses for inactivity, but check with your doctor before starting an exercise program—especially if you're over 30, overweight, have been sedentary for several years, are a heavy smoker, use alcohol or drugs, or have any medical problems. Start slowly the low-stress way room facilities, you have no problem. Otherwise you may have to keep a washcloth and towel at work and use the company restroom to "freshen up." If you take a shower before leaving home, any perspiration you excrete will be clean sweat from a healthy workout. Malodorous perspiration occurs from sweating during periods of anxiety. Your bike rides will become relaxing.

Keep a change of clothes at work, or carry it with you. If you have a short commute on level terrain, wear your work clothes, using a pants clip on your right leg. Otherwise you should wear comfortable cycling clothes appropriate for the climate. Clean clothes can be tucked away at work, and social clothes retrieved on a day when you drive. Carry your briefcase or purse in special bicycle bags or tie them carefully to racks on the back of your bike.

You could also wear a knapsack, but if it is heavy, it could cause some lower back stress. It also can create problems with stability because it raises your center of gravity.

Plan Your Route—Commuting by bike requires some planning and ingenuity. Map out the course you plan to take and test it on a day off. You may have to take a different route than you normally travel to avoid freeways and congested roads.

Some things to keep in mind are: low traffic, width and smoothness of streets, hills, busy intersections, directness and safety. It may be worthwhile to follow a little longer route if it provides you with better scenery and safety. After all, the idea is to combine pleasure, low-stress exercise and practicality.

When you drive the course, make note of different landmarks and the distance or mileage to reach them. Take the test ride with whatever you would normally carry. The idea is to time the commute, taking it easy. If you're doing your test ride on a weekend, you may have to allow a little extra time for traffic at intersections. Cars move slowly in congested streets, and a bicyclist can often move faster than cars in those circumstances.

Time Estimates—You can pedal at 8 miles per hour even if you are in mediocre physical condition. You will find that as you get in better shape your speeds will increase. A ride that takes 40 minutes today will take 30 minutes in a month or so. Each day you will cut a minute or two off your time. Remember to go slowly and easily at first, being very careful of traffic.

It's a good idea to start out trying the commute just one or two days a week. Check the weather conditions and plan your rides on days that promise to be pleasant.

The Exercise Plan—Map out some pleasant, safe routes for your cycling workout. Try to select streets that are relatively traffic-free. Use your car to measure miles, then make a note of a landmark at each mile.

Variety is important to prevent boredom, so it's good to have several routes. Venture off on your bike over a possible route, then go back in the car

BICYCLING WORKOUT
(Beginner Level)

Week	Miles	Time (min.)
1	1	Comfortable pace
2	2	Comfortable pace
3	2	11
4	3	16
5	3	15
6	4	24
7	4	23
8	5	28
9	5	26
10	6	36
11	6	35
12	7	42

BICYCLING WORKOUT
(Intermediate Level)

Week	Miles	Time (min.)
1	8	50
2	8	45
3	8	42
4	9	56
5	9	54
6	10	62
7	10	60
8	10	55
9	11	63
10	11	60
11	12	68
12	12	62

A LOW-STRESS BICYCLING CHAMPION

At 89, Fred Knoller is my kind of low-stress cyclist. Because of his age, he often goes unchallenged in competition, but that doesn't mean he is a softie. Fred is the oldest competitor of the U.S. Cycling Federation.

He passed his 50th year in bicycling a few years ago at the U.S. Cycling Federation 1980 national championships in Bisbee, Arizona. He said then that exercise and good food kept him young.

At his home in Florida, Knoller keeps up a regular fitness routine: He rides 20 miles three times a week, works out with light weights, does calisthenics, takes two-mile walks along the beach, goes to dances twice a week, stands on his head for five minutes at a time and easily executes 10 pullups during workouts. His diet includes lots of raw, leafy vegetables and not much meat.

Knoller caught "cycling fever" at Madison Square Garden in 1914 when he watched riders circle the board track during a six-day race. The high point of his own career came in 1949 when, at the age of 53, he won the German Bike Club's 100-mile handicapped race. He won that race in 4 hours and 14 minutes, an incredibly swift time for a 53-year-old.

Into his mature years, he continues to enter races. During the championship race in Bisbee a few years back, he was hit by another rider and crashed to the pavement just three miles from the finish line. Battered and bruised, he fixed his bike, continued on and finished the race. Asked why he didn't wait to ride the ambulance back in, Knoller answered, "If you don't finish, you don't win a prize. I would have picked up the bike and run with it to finish."

Fred Knoller keeps on rolling!

(Material adapted from a *Tucson Citizen* article by Ed Stiles.)

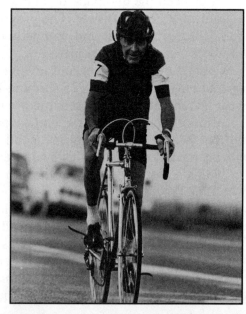

and measure the distance. One of my favorite routes has a beautiful area where I can add extra miles by repeating a loop. I think that bicycling will soon become one of your favorite sports.

LOW-STRESS SWIMMING PLAN

Once your fears are tamed, techniques become natural and relaxed. Your new habits let you focus less on your body's action. Swimming becomes a tranquil activity as your body takes over the physical movements, and your mind indulges in self-exploration, creativity and mental satisfaction.

Lap Swimming—Before learning to swim again, I could never understand how people could swim lap after lap in pools. But now, having mastered swimming, I know the satisfaction and security they experience.

When I began to swim laps I bumped into a few swimmers and had some embarrassing moments until I learned "lap-swim etiquette." Pools often designate specific times for lap swimming and divide the pool into lanes. There will be areas for slow, medium and fast swimmers. If they aren't marked, ask the lifeguard which is which. Unless you're a very good swimmer, avoid the fast lanes.

Warmup—Always start your swim with a slow warmup and finish with a slow cool-down. The best place for this is in the slower lanes. The slow lane should also be your choice if you are working out with a kickboard or other training device.

Masters Swim—If you have a competitive nature, enjoy swimming with others, or need the discipline of an organized workout, the Masters Swimming Program may be the answer. The program began in 1970 to promote physical fitness through training and competitive swimming. Now more than 15,000 swimmers nationwide participate.

Competition is low-key and involves swimmers at all levels of ability. Participants range in age from 25 through 85. They compete in groups set off by 5-year increments. Training sessions are usually held several times a week.

A lot of members don't even take part in the competitive meets. Still, they find that joining the program is a good way to improve their swimming while enjoying the fellowship of other swimmers.

If this sounds interesting, you can get more information on the Masters Swimming Program from:

USMS Office, c/o Dorothy Donnelly, 5 Piggot Lane, Avon, CT 06001. Be sure to include a self-addressed, stamped envelope. Or, call (203) 677-9464.

The Exercise Plan—The plan I've designed is based on a 25-yard pool, the average size of many indoor pools. Ask the lifeguard the length of the pool you will be using. If the pool is longer or shorter, adjust the information in the tables accordingly. Your progress may be quicker or slower than the suggested workouts, but they can serve as a guide in setting goals. Learn to be your own coach.

WALKING/BIKING/SWIMMING COMBINATION

The forms on the next two pages show how you can combine all of the low-stress exercises—walking, biking and swimming—in a weekly workout. Notice that I alternate an easy workout with a hard workout. Use the "rest day" when you're feeling particularly worn out.

Copy the blank form on page 175 and use it to record your progress each week. Reviewing your charts and comments can help you determine your own best times to work out.

SWIMMING WORKOUT
(Beginner Level)

Week	Rests	Repetitions	Distance	Total Laps*
1-2	When needed	4 laps	100 yds	4
3-4	End of each lap	4x25 yds	100 yds	4
5-6	End of each lap	8x25 yds	200 yds	8
7-8	End of 2 laps	4x50 yds	200 yds	8
9-10	End of 3 laps	3x75 yds	225 yds	9
11-12	End of 3 laps	3x100 yds	300 yds	12

*Based on a 25-yd pool.

SWIMMING WORKOUT
(Intermediate Level)

Week	Rests	Repetitions	Distance	Total Laps*
1-2	End of 4 laps	2x100 yds	200 yds	8
3-4	End of 3 laps	4x75 yds	300 yds	12
5-6	End of 4 laps	3x100 yds	300 yds	12
7-8	End of 2 laps	8x50 yds	400 yds	16
9-10	End of 4 laps	4x100 yds	400 yds	16
11-12	End of 4 laps	5x100 yds	500 yds	20

*Based on a 25-yd pool.

At the bottom of the form is a place to record your weight. When weighing yourself each week, try to do it at the same time each day, preferably morning. Add up your weekly miles for each sport and the time spent on exercise. Be proud of yourself for improving your health.

YOUR COMMITMENT

Start today with your own dream and commitment to walk around the block, take a dip in the pool, or pedal a bike. Stretch your body and your horizons.

Make and keep your exercise program relaxed and non-stressful. Who knows where it may lead! You might find me alongside you in a triathlon sometime during the next 40 years.

Meanwhile, good luck and good health!

WEEKLY WORKOUT

Day	Date	Exercise	Time (min.)	Distance	Intensity	Comments
Sunday noon	5/6	Stretch/Walk Bike Stretch	15 40 10	 7.5 miles	 Hard	Outdoor stretch—fun! Shifting getting easier.
Monday	5/7	Rest			Easy	
Tuesday p.m.	5/8	Stretch Swim Stretch	20 20 20	 300 yds	 Hard	Aggressive swimming. Peaceful stretch.
Wednesday a.m.	5/9	Stretch Walk	10 50	 3 miles	 Easy	Solved problem. Tranquil walk.
Thursday p.m.	5/10	Stretch Bike Walk	15 20 30	 4 miles 2 miles	 Intermediate	Biked to Jill's and walked with her.
Friday a.m.	5/11	Stretch Bike	20 30	 6 miles	 Hard	Increased mph.
Saturday a.m.	5/12	Stretch Swim Stretch	15 30 15	 350 yds	 Intermediate	Slow start; but felt great afterward.

Weight: 112 lbs.

Total Exercise Time: 6 hours
Swimming: 650 yds
Biking: 17.5 miles
Walking: 5 miles

WEEKLY WORKOUT

Day	Date	Exercise	Time (min.)	Distance	Intensity	Comments
Sunday						
Monday						
Tuesday						
Wednesday						
Thursday						
Friday						
Saturday						

Weight: _____

Total Exercise Time: _____
Swimming: _____
Biking: _____
Walking: _____

Index

METRIC EQUIVALENTS

yds.	miles	meters
25	0.01	23
50	0.03	46
100	0.06	91
1000	0.57	914
1760	1.0	1609
2640	1.5	2414
3520	2.0	3219